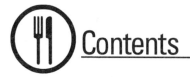 Contents

Introduction 5

Chapter 1:
Everything You Ever Wanted to Ask
Your Doctor About Breast Cancer... 9

Chapter 2:
The Diet and Breast Cancer Connection 22

Chapter 3:
Everything You Ever Wanted to Ask
a Dietitian About Preventing Breast Cancer... 36

Chapter 4:
The 10 Food Steps to Freedom 45

Chapter 5:
The Joy of Eating 79

Chapter 6:
The Recipes You Cannot Live Without 90

Chapter 7:
Navigating the Supermarket 127

Chapter 8:
Restaurant Rules to Live By 144

Index 155

Tell Me What to Eat to Help Prevent Breast Cancer

Nutrition You Can Live With

by

Elaine Magee, MPH, RD

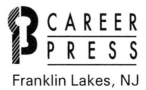

CAREER
PRESS

Franklin Lakes, NJ

TELL ME WHAT TO EAT TO HELP PREVENT BREAST CANCER
Cover design by Lu Rossman
Printed in the U.S.A. by Book-mart Press

To order this title, please call toll-free 1-800-CAREER-1 (NJ and Canada:
201-848-0310) to order using VISA or MasterCard, or for further information on
books from Career Press.

The Career Press, Inc., 3 Tice Road, PO Box 687, Franklin Lakes, NJ 07417
www.careerpress.com

Library of Congress Cataloging-in-Publication Data

Magee, Elaine.
    Tell me what to eat to help prevent breast cancer / by Elaine Magee.
        p.   cm.
    Includes index.
    ISBN 1-56414-447-X (paper)
    1. Breast—Cancer—Diet therapy. 2. Breast—Cancer—Prevention. I. Title.

RC280.B8 M255 2000
616.99'449052—dc21   00-020749

Introduction

As I approach my 40s, I am probably most afraid of having ovarian or breast cancer. I have heart disease in my family tree so I've always paid attention to the research on heart disease prevention. But if you ask me what disease I am most fearful of at this point in my life, I would choose breast cancer, hands down. I do happen to live in what I call "the buckle" of the breast cancer belt—The San Franciso Bay area, which has one of the highest rates of breast cancer in the country.

Granted, I have a few things feeding this particular fear. My mother is a breast cancer survivor. She was diagnosed in her late 50s and underwent a modified radical mastectomy (removal of the entire breast and some of the underarm lymph nodes) along with six months of chemotherapy.

At many of the "Women and Heart Disease" conferences I have attended, the keynote speakers almost always ask the audience why they are so afraid of breast cancer—most of them will be struck down by heart disease. They always have impressive statistics to cite as well. Of course, all of that is true; many women will eventually die of heart disease...but usually in our later years (after menopause).

What these speakers don't realize is that many of us, in our younger years, have already witnessed friends and family members in their 30s, 40s, and 50s battle breast cancer. I don't personally know of any woman who had heart disease before having the chance to marry, have children, or complete life goals.

It is said that every three minutes a woman in the United States learns she has breast cancer (*FDA Consumer*, July 1999). Next to skin cancer, breast cancer is the most common cancer among women—second only to lung cancer in cancer deaths in women. While it is true that three out of four women who have been diagnosed with breast cancer are age 50 or older, I have also read that breast cancer is more aggressive in younger women. You better believe young women are fearful of breast cancer—we have every right to be.

Being cautiously optimistic

Some women think that if you have breast cancer in your family, you are doomed. Actually, only 5 percent of breast cancer cases are due to a genetic predisposition. So what makes up the rest of the risk? At least 50 percent of breast cancer cases may be "explained" by known or suspected risk factors, which include things you can change in your lifestyle (what you eat, being overweight, exercising regularly, using alcohol, etc.). You'll find these potentially beneficial lifestyle changes in "The 10 Food Steps to Freedom" in Chapter 4.

But understand that many researchers feel we don't have scientific proof that eating or avoiding certain foods can prevent breast cancer. (For example, some of the groundbreaking research has been done on female rats—not women). And the long-term effects of the foods that are currently being suggested by some as potential food helpers haven't been fully studied (such as eating more soy or supplementing your diet with flaxseed).

Most of all, researchers are afraid that if people start taking certain food steps to help prevent breast cancer, they might stop taking other important steps (such as breast self-exam, having mammograms, avoiding tobacco, and so forth).

I'm expecting that because you are concerned about helping yourself prevent breast cancer, you will maintain your annual appointments with your OB/GYN, keep to your mammogram schedule, and perform monthly self-exams. You will also probably want to take a good look at "The 10 Food Steps to Freedom" in this book, incorporating as many steps as you can. You will feel good doing this because they all benefit your overall health. At the same time, they help prevent other chronic diseases such as heart disease, osteoporosis, type-II diabetes, and obesity.

There is some good news

Not that there is ever a good time to be diagnosed with breast cancer, but women diagnosed with it today have more effective treatment options and much more reason to be optimistic about their recovery than the women before them. This is thanks to new drugs, new procedures, advances in research, and better diagnostic techniques.

For example, a new procedure called sentinel node biopsy (still under investigation) allows physicians to pinpoint the first lymph node into which a tumor drains, and potentially enables them to remove only the nodes likely to contain cancer cells. In addition, the FDA has recently approved several new drugs and new uses for older drugs. Some of these are thought to improve the chances of successfully treating breast cancer and one is known to help cancer patients with severe pain. And, according to the American Cancer Society, breast cancer death rates are going down. That might be the best news of all!

Turn your fear into action

We can't do anything about some risk factors of breast cancer (such as our genetics or the ages we started menstruating, had our children, or went through menopause). But we can try to tip the scales in our favor by taking some common-sense lifestyle steps.

Listen, we may not have all the evidence about how food and nutrients play a role in preventing breast cancer, but we do have some clues. This book puts our best clues together and works them into 10 food and lifestyle steps that you will be able to follow. This book isn't called *Eat This and You'll Never Have to Worry About Breast Cancer* or *This is the Answer You've Been Waiting for*...it simply looks at the evidence thus far and answers the question, "Tell me what to eat to help prevent breast cancer."

 Chapter 1

Everything You Ever Wanted to Ask Your Doctor About Breast Cancer...

Questions about *getting* breast cancer

Isn't it just a matter of chance whether you get or don't get cancer?

The answer to this question is bittersweet. Some scientists believe that more than 80 percent of all cancers are associated with a few lifestyle factors we can control:

- Diet.
- Smoking.
- Exposure to the sun.
  (American Institute for Cancer Research)

That's the "sweet" part. The "bitter" part arises when people then blame themselves if they get cancer, thinking it was their fault in some way.

We still don't know the whole story about cancer and we can't predict who will get it. Perhaps the best way to look at this is to do the best you can to put the odds in your favor by living the most healthy lifestyle you can.

Percentages of Cancer Deaths Attributed to Various Factors

Diet	35 percent
Tobacco	30 percent
Occupation	4 percent
Radon	2 to 3 percent
Pollution	2 percent
Medical X-rays	0.5 percent

To help you, the American Institute for Cancer Research published the table above to help paint a picture of what you can do to reduce your risk of cancer. In addition:

- Women whose closest female relatives (mothers or sisters or daughters) have had breast cancer—the risk increases if her relative's cancer developed before menopause or if it affected both breasts.
- Women who started menstruating before age 12 or had a late menopause (after age 55).
- Women who have never had children or had their first child after age 30.
- Women who have already had breast cancer are at the highest risk.

Looking at who is at risk from a global perspective, North American women are at an increased risk for breast cancer compared to other parts of the world.

Q **Am I at an increased risk for breast cancer if I have fibrocystic breast tissue?**

There is no evidence that fibrocystic breast disease, fibrocystic tissue, or benign changes in breast tissues (such as atypical hyperplasia) are associated with cancer. Having fibrocystic breast tissue might make finding other lumps more difficult. It is very important to keep up with your monthly self breast exams, your annual appointments with your practitioner, and follow-ups with your doctor on any lumps that are found and tested to be aware if they were considered the precancerous type.

Q **Is there anything I can do if I have fibrocystic breast disease?**

You may not be able to prevent fibrocystic breast disease, but you may be able to reduce the symptoms. Although it hasn't been proven, avoiding caffeine and chocolate may decrease the symptoms. A low-sodium diet has also been suggested in helping in the second half of the menstrual cycle.

Q **Are breast cancer rates increasing or decreasing?**

According to data from the Connecticut Tumor Registry, the incidence of invasive breast cancer hasn't changed much since 1990. However, we are detecting more and more cancers in their first stages and fewer in the more advanced stages (*Connecticut Medicine,* January 1999).

Q **At what age are we most at risk for breast cancer?**

Generally, the older we are, the higher our risk of breast cancer becomes. About 5 percent of breast cancer patients are under the age of 40. But the younger we are, the more fatal the breast cancer tends to be. It's actually the leading cause of cancer death among women between the ages of 15 and 54. (Take a look at the chart on page 12 for more information.)

A one-in-nine lifetime risk of getting breast cancer is rather frightening. However, this statistic includes people in their 90s as well as those in their 30s. The National Cancer Institute calculates the risk for women under 35 years as one in 622. They increase the risk to one in 93 by age 45 and one in 33 by age 55. By age 65 the risk is one in 17.

Breast Cancer's Toll

Projected 1996 cases:	184,300
Number who will die:	44,300
Current U.S. survivors:	2 million
Lifetime risk, 1996:	1 in 9
Lifetime risk, 1960:	1 in 14

(**Source:** *National Alliance of Breast Cancer Organizations*)

How does breast cancer start?

All breast cancers share a defect in the DNA or genetic code that normally regulates cell division. One of three things happens:

- There is accelerated cell growth.
- There isn't any braking mechanism to slow it down.
- The DNA repair mechanism is not working.

Thousands of times every day a healthy body takes care of cancer-like aberrations. It is possible that cancer begins when our normal regulatory breakdowns go unrepaired by our bodies.

Cancer does not occur due to a single event, but is a process that may take two decades or more to develop. Cancer risk rises with regular exposure to carcinogens over many years.

There are three major stages in cancer development:

1. **Initiation:** Cancer-causing agents damage a cell's genetic material.
2. **Promotion:** Damaged cells are exposed to chemicals that speed up cell division. Long-term exposure to these promoters is necessary for cancer to develop. Nutritional factors are thought to have their greatest contribution on cancer in this stage.
3. **Progression** Cells become fully malignant and acquire the ability to metastasize (or spread) to other parts of the body.

We know that a cancerous lump's genesis is a long process containing a series of biological events that drove a normal breast cell towards cancerous growth. But we do not know when the initiation of breast cancer occurs and why.

It takes one billion cancer cells to make a one-centimeter tumor. Researchers believe that cancer may grow for as long as eight years before being detected by an X-ray.

Some researchers believe that at least 50 percent of breast cancer may be "explained" by known or suspected risk factors, including things you can change (what you eat, being over-weight, not exercising regularly, and alcohol use [*Connecticut Medicine*, January, 1999]).

To what organs does breast cancer tend to spread?
Breast tumor cells, over time, can circulate through the blood and lymphatic systems and start growing in other organs (usually the liver, lungs, or bones).

How much do your genes or family history change your risk?
About 5 percent of women with breast cancer have a hereditary form of this disease. These women usually develop breast cancer before menopause and have several family members with the disease as well. One way this genetic risk is detected is by measuring mutations on two particular genes (BRCA1 and BRCA2). However, this controversial genetic test can only tell you if you are more likely to develop breast cancer. It can not assure you that you will never get it, considering the majority of breast cancer cases aren't hereditary.

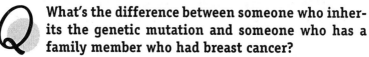

What's the difference between someone who inherits the genetic mutation and someone who has a family member who had breast cancer?
Researchers are still working on the answer to this question. Your risk is thought to be higher if you inherit the genetic mutation, compared to just having a family history of

breast cancer. But if a first-degree relative (mother, sister, or daughter) has breast cancer—especially before age 40—your risk is also increased.

Q **What about those new genetic tests?**
Genetic testing (along with the inevitable consequences for women whom test positive for the BRCA gene mutations) are still being worked through. Many researchers feel that genetic testing should take place only as part of a clinical research study so women can have access to psychological assistance and follow-ups.

Q **Where in the United States are breast cancer rates highest?**
Long Island (NY), the San Francisco area, and some areas around the Great Lakes have higher rates of breast cancer than the rest of the country.

Q **What are the other risk factors for breast cancer?**
Before you look through the list below keep two things in mind: 75 percent of all breast cancers are found in women over 50 and 75 percent occur in women not considered high-risk. Obviously there is still a lot more we don't know about breast cancer.

Breast cancer is known to develop at a higher rate among women who:
- Get their first period before age 12.
- Reach menopause later (after 55).
- Are late in childbearing (having a first child after age 30 or being childless altogether).
- Do not breast feed.
- Are obese (30 percent or more above "ideal" weight, according to age, sex, and height).

The above criteria are thought to increase or prolong levels of circulating estrogen in women's bodies. For example, when you are pregnant or breastfeeding the production of estrogen is interrupted.

Some other potential risk factors still being investigated (some of which are still considered controversial):

- Abnormal biopsy (women who have had abnormal or precancerous cells in breast lumps, such as cysts or fibroadenomas).
- Exposure to cigarette smoke.
- The use of oral contraceptives or hormone replacement therapy.
- Induced abortion.
- Exercise levels.
- Exposure to pesticides.

 What is the latest information on hormone replacement therapy (for perimenopause) and breast cancer risk?

Even though we know there is this link between higher levels of estrogen in our bodies and an increased risk of breast cancer, there still doesn't seem to be conclusive research on breast cancer and hormone replacement therapy. One large Harvard study now suggests that women who have been on HRT for more than 10 years have an increased risk of dying from breast cancer. And if that isn't confusing enough, women who take HRT for less than 10 years might actually have a decreased risk.

One hypothesis is that a high estrogenic environment during the perinatal period increases breast cancer risk for girl babies later in their adult lives. Some researchers suspect that a mother's intake of fats during pregnancy may increase the risk of breast cancer in daughters.

Over the last 25 years, more than 50 studies have examined the possible relationship between HRT and breast cancer. Some have shown an increased risk and some have not. Many researchers believe there is little or no increased risk of breast cancer when HRT is used for 10 years or less.

It may all come down to each woman and her doctor or nurse practitioner weighing her own personal risk factors for heart disease, osteoporosis, and cancer, and to the severity of her menopausal symptoms when it comes time to decide whether to use hormone replacement therapy.

Questions about finding breast cancer

Q **What is the best way to find breast cancer?**
Currently, the most effective technique for early detection is mammography. Mammography is a low-dose X-ray procedure that can detect small tumors and breast abnormalities up to two years before they can be found by touch. The earlier a tumor in the breast is found, the more treatable it is and the more likely the patient is to survive. It's not surprising that regular mammograms decrease the chance of dying from breast cancer.

What about regular breast self-examinations? It is still a good idea to check your breasts for lumps or anything abnormal—just to be sure. You might be getting a mammogram every year or every other year and self-examination is something you can do in between. Anything you can do to catch a tumor sooner is worth the effort. Have your doctor or nurse practitioner conduct a clinical breast exam during your annual gynecological exam. If they haven't been doing it automatically every year, ask them to—it's very important.

Q **Are lumps the only warning signs of breast cancer?**
No. Not all breast cancers form lumps. The following are all possible warning signs of breast cancer. If you detect any of them, please see your practitioner immediately:

- A lump or a thickening in or near the breast or in the underarm area.
- A change in breast size or shape.
- A discharge from the nipple (although cancer is rarely the cause).
- Retraction of the nipple.
- A change in skin color or feel of the skin of the breast, areolas, or nipples (dimpled, puckered, or scaly).
- Swelling, redness, or heat in the breast.

Q **When is the best time to do your breast self-exam?**
The best time to do your monthly breast self-exam tends to be a few days after your menstrual period has ended when your breasts are not tender or swollen. If you no longer have a period due to a hysterectomy (but you still have your ovaries), use the tenderness or swelling of your breasts as your guide. Notice when your breasts are tender, then do your breast self-exam a few days after the tenderness has ended. If you have already gone through menopause make a habit of checking your breasts the same time every month (such as the first of every month).

Q **I've heard mammograms don't work as well in younger women. Is that true?**
The dense young breast is often difficult to "image" on a mammogram—the picture actually appears cloudy. But as the breast ages, more and more fatty tissue replaces the dense tissue and the fat tissue shows up clearly in mammograms. This is one reason why routine mammograms aren't recommended for women under age 40 (other than a baseline mammogram). It has been reported that mammograms miss between 10 and 15 percent of all breast cancers in women under 50.

Q **How often should I get a mammogram and when should I start?**
While the experts continue to debate this hot topic, the National Cancer Institute recommends women in their 40s have mammograms every one to two years. The American Cancer Society encourages yearly mammograms because breast cancer can grow faster in women under 50. In this case, catching a tumor early can be of vital importance.

Most experts agree it's a good idea to go ahead and have a baseline mammogram between the ages of 35 and 40 so there can be a record of what was "normal" for you at this age and it can be compared to mammograms performed at later ages. Some researchers have even suggested having your first mammogram 10 years before the age of the person in your family who had breast cancer. So if your mother or aunt had breast cancer at the age of 45, you might consider getting a mammogram at 35.

Q Do most breast lumps tend to be cancer?
About 80 percent of breast lumps are benign (not cancerous). But any lump you or your doctor finds should be checked out as soon as possible just in case it is.

Questions about breast cancer tumors

Q I've heard of fast- and slow-growing breast cancer. What does this mean?
Slow-growing breast tumors, about 25 percent of all cases, tend to be the most curable because they usually don't spread and they are more likely to be detected on a mammogram than during a clinical or self breast exam.

Moderate-growth tumors account for about 50 percent of all breast cancers and are also very treatable. They are picked up by mammograms and clinical and/or self-breast exams.

This leaves us with the more aggressive, fast-growing tumors. For a variety of potential reasons (genetic predisposition or a higher level of estrogen) these tumors spread more rapidly in premenopausal women. What is most dangerous about this type of tumor is that it may spread before it's picked up by a mammogram or a clinical and/or self-breast exam.

Q What is Stage I, II, or III breast cancer?
The stage of the breast cancer refers to the size of a tumor and how far the cancer has spread within the breast, to nearby tissues, and to other organs. The following are the general descriptions of the various stages:

- **Carcinoma In Situ:** Cancer is confined to milk-producing glands or ducts (passages connecting the glands to the nipple) and has not invaded nearby breast tissue.
- **Stage I:** The tumor is smaller than or equal to two centimeters in diameter and underarm lymph nodes test negative for cancer.

- **Stage II:** The tumor is larger than two centimeters in diameter and lymph nodes test negative for cancer, or the tumor is less than or equal to five centimeters with lymph nodes testing positive for cancer.

- **Stage IIIA:** The tumor is larger than five centimeters with lymph nodes testing positive for breast cancer, or the tumor is any size with lymph nodes that stick to one another or surrounding tissue.

- **Stage IIIB:** When the tumor of any size has spread to the skin, chest wall, or internal mammary lymph nodes, which are located beneath the breast and inside the chest.

- **Stage IV:** When the tumor of any size has spread (metastasized) to distant sites, such as the bones, lungs, or lymph nodes away from the breasts.

How effective is treating breast cancer today?
Although treatment is initially successful for many women, the American Cancer Society estimates that breast cancer tends to return in approximately 50 percent of these cases.

What are the types of treatment available to women today?
Breast cancer can be treated with one or a combination of the following:

- **Surgery.** (Most women with breast cancer will have some type of surgery, depending on the stage of the breast cancer.)
- **Radiation.**
- **Drugs** (chemotherapy and hormonal therapy).

Can you explain the big words associated with breast cancer?
Here's a partial list of the words you need to know concerning breast cancer:

- **Axillary lymph nodes:** Bean-shaped glands under the arm that help fight infection.

- **Calcifications:** Tiny calcium deposits that resemble grains of salt on a mammogram.
- **Ducts:** Tubes in the breast that carry milk from the lobules to the nipple.
- **Estrogen:** The female sex hormone produced in the ovaries, adrenal glands, fat, and placenta.
- **Hormonal therapy:** Drug therapy that prevents natural hormones from stimulating cancer cells. For example, Tamoxifen is an estrogen blocker and aromatase inhibitor that blocks the production of estrogen in the body.
- **Lobules:** The part of the breast that makes breast milk.
- **Lumpectomy:** Breast-conserving surgery that removes a lump or a layer of surrounding tissue.
- **Mastectomy:** Surgical removal of the entire breast.
- **Metastasis:** The spread of cancer through the blood or lymphatic system to other sites.
- **Oncogenes:** Genes that cause normal cells to become cancerous.
- **Palpate:** To examine the breast by touch.
- **Stem cells:** "Naïve" cells in the bone marrow and blood that eventually produce mature red and white blood cells and platelets.

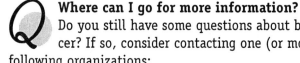 **Where can I go for more information?**
Do you still have some questions about breast cancer? If so, consider contacting one (or more) of the following organizations:

- **American Cancer Society**
  (800)ACS-2345
  www.cancer.org

- **American Institute for Cancer Research**
  (800)843-8114
  www.aicr.org
  E-mail: aicrweb@aicr.org

- **CancerNet**
  www.icic.nci.nih.gov
- **CancerCenter**
  www.cancercenter.com
- **National Alliance of Breast Cancer Organizations**
  (800)719-9154
  www.nabco.org
- **National Cancer Institute**
  (800)4-CANCER
  www.nci.nih.gov
- **Y-Me National Breast Cancer Hotline**
  (800)221-2141
  www.y-me.org
- **University of Pennsylvania Cancer Center**
  (800)789-PENN
  www.oncolink.upenn.edu

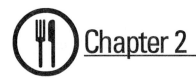 Chapter 2

The Diet and Breast Cancer Connection

I t has been estimated by studies in the 1980s and 90s that about 35 percent of all cancer deaths are attributable to diet. Approximately 40 percent of all cancer in men and about 60 percent of all cancers in women are associated with diet (American Institute for Cancer Research, 1992). The trouble is that the actual roles of particular foods and the amounts that either cause or help prevent cancer are still not clear.

However, it appears that a diet rich in vegetables, fruits, and whole grains helps protect against cancer, while too much fat—both saturated and certain types of unsaturated—and alcohol seem to increase the risk of developing a number of cancers. We are starting to know more about the specific components in foods that have anticancer properties. Fruits and vegetables, for example, are loaded with them.

Why is finding the "proof" so difficult?

Many major studies draw their conclusions by comparing how large population groups eat, and their health, with other groups'. We conduct laboratory studies on rats, but what happens to rats in the lab is not always the same thing that happens to humans living their normal lives. These studies can give us some clues. They give links and associations that are definitely helpful...but they are not considered proof of a cause/effect relationship.

The medical establishment still hasn't put its stamp of approval on dietary theories of cancer cause and/or prevention. *The Journal of the National Cancer Institute* states: "Much attention has focused on possible dietary means of lowering breast cancer risk, but most studies to date have yielded inconclusive findings."

Dr. Robert Russell of the USDA Human Nutrition Research Center at Tufts University says that "flaxseed, garlic, fish oil, and soy are all unproved in terms of reducing risk of breast cancer." He adds that a diet low in fat and high in fruits and vegetables might possibly reduce risk.

However, the only way to get this proof is to hold a large, scientifically controlled study that carefully monitors the diets of

---

F.Y.I. Looking back over the past 40 years

- **1960s:** Research suggested that diet had a major role in the development of many cancers and that limiting certain foods might play a part in cancer prevention.
- **1970s:** Scientists estimated that diet contributed to cancer deaths in as many as 40 percent of the cases in men and 60 percent in women.
- **1980s:** Another statistic was released: 35 percent of cancer deaths were said to be related to certain elements in the diet.
- **1990s:** We've learned more and collected more information about the relationship between what we eat and cancer risk, but we still don't have the proof of prevention in our hands.

humans, noting the diseases they develop over their lives. These studies are obviously very expensive and may take decades to show results. Can we wait that long? I can't. I think we have enough clues right now to take some educated guesses. Each step is healthy to do anyway (for your heart, your bones, your energy level, and so forth) so why not talk about them now?

Fat and cancer

Although there is lots of research on dietary fat and cancer, there is still no definitive proof that dietary fat encourages cancer. Yet there is no question that population groups with a high fat intake also have higher cancer rates. Population studies between America and Japan have shown a strong correlation between fat and cancer—especially in the breast, colon, prostate, rectum, and lining of the uterus. Most research indicates that the total amount of dietary fat is important, while some newer studies suggest that type of fat might also be important.

Selenium and cancer

Various forms of selenium have demonstrated the ability to kill cancer cells and limit their ability to multiply in animal models. The selenium metabolite methylselenol was three to four times more effective in killing certain cells and avoiding harmful DNA breaks than other selenium compounds tested. It acts to prevent the formation of, and reduce the multiplication of, blood vessels surrounding cancerous cells by starving the cancer to death. (Dr. Junxuan Lu, scientist at the AMC Cancer Research Center in Denver, Colorado). Researchers discovered that patients with certain cancers had very low levels of selenium. Where do we get selenium (not counting our multivitamins)? It can be found in whole grains, legumes, Brazil nuts, seafood, lean meats, eggs, and fruits and vegetables grown in selenium-rich soil.

Tea polyphenol and cancer

Tea polyphenol is one of the few agents that appears to affect carcinogens at the stages of initiation, promotion, and progression. The cancer-inhibiting powers of tea have been amply demonstrated in animal and human cell line studies. The next step is seeing if such inhibitory effects apply to humans and then at what concentrations. (Dr. Chung S. Yang, professor Rutgers University Dept. of Chemical Biology and college of Pharmacy, Piscataway, New Jersey).

It's all in the estrogen?

So is breast cancer all about our estrogen levels? So far, some animal studies show that during pregnancy, high amounts of corn oil (which contains mainly the more undesirable omega-6 fatty acids) increases estrogen levels (estradiol) during pregnancy and increases the risk of breast cancer among the female rat offspring (*Nutrition*, May, 1999).

Recent studies indicate that a high level of estrogen may be a major risk factor for developing uterine (endometrial) cancer. There is a study going on right now at the University of Hawaii Cancer Research Center in Honolulu studying the correlation between diet and uterine cancer risk. One of their researchers, Marc

---

F.Y.I. Phytochemicals

Phytochemicals (plant compounds or chemicals) may help prevent tumors in three ways:

1. They have antioxidant properties.
2. They help activate (turn on) carcinogen-detoxifying enzymes.
3. They help inhibit tumor cell proliferation (rapid increasing).

Goodman, Ph.D., thinks fat in food and on the body may have a direct effect on circulating levels of estrogen—because body fat produces estrogen. So far data from their center suggest that diets low in calories and rich in produce, whole grains, and legumes (especially soybeans) can reduce the risk of uterine cancer.

Produce and breast cancer

I think we all know that fruits and vegetables (full of important vitamins, minerals, fiber, and phytochemicals) are healthy and wouldn't be surprised to hear that they help reduce our risk of most cancers. In fact, for most of my adult life I have seen this same statistic: A poor diet (lacking in fruits, vegetables, and whole grains) may be responsible for one-third of *all* cancer cases worldwide. Some of the vitamins, minerals, and phytochemicals in fruits and vegetables act as antioxidants to inhibit at least one step in the cancer process—damage to DNA.

What is an antioxidant?

An antioxidant is any substance that, when present at low concentrations, compared to those of an oxidizable substrate (such as proteins, lipids, or carbohydrates), significantly delays or prevents oxidation of that substrate. These substances protect against oxygen damage by neutralizing the harmful effects of free radicals. Free radicals are produced by normal body processes and common external hazards (such as ultraviolet light, X-rays and other radiation, heat, cigarette smoke, alcohol, and some pollutants.) The U.S. Food and Drug Administration recognizes four food-based antioxidants: vitamin C, vitamin E, vitamin A (precursor to beta carotene), and selenium.

The carotenoids (the phytochemical family that includes beta carotene) are known to reduce oxidative DNA damage and stimulate the immune system, which helps prevent cancer. You will find the carotenoids and vitamin C primarily in fruits and vegetables.

But what about breast cancer? Can produce or certain kinds of fruits and vegetables help reduce our risk of breast cancer? Researchers recently looked at the long-term intakes of vitamins A, C, and E and fruits and vegetables and breast cancer rates with data from the big "Nurses' Health Study" done by the National Institutes of Health (tracking 89,494 women for eight years). The most encouraging results were for premenopausal women. Premenopausal women who ate five or more servings per day of fruits and vegetables had a modestly lower risk of breast cancer (compared to those who ate fewer than two servings per day). Intakes of beta carotene from food and supplements and vitamin A from foods were weakly associated with a reduction in breast cancer risk (even after adjusting for age, total calories, age at menarche [first menstrual period], family history of breast cancer, alcohol intake and body mass index [percentage of weight vs. fat in relation to height] at age 18).

Antioxidant vitamins, carotenoids, and breast cancer

Many researchers have suspected a link between antioxidants, the carotenoids, and breast cancer but so far the studies have been inconclusive. Perhaps we needed to look at their effect (in food) on breast cancer in premenopausal women only.

A recent study gives some encouraging results. Harvard researchers looked at the data for 2,697 women with invasive breast cancer (784 premenopausal and 1,913 postmenopausal). They found an association between higher food intakes of alpha and beta carotene, lutein/zeaxanithin, vitamin C, and vitamin A with lower breast cancer risk—particularly among premenopausal women with a family history of breast cancer. They also looked at fruit and vegetable intake in general and found the premenopausal women who ate five or more servings a day had a modestly lower risk of breast cancer than those who ate fewer than two servings per day. Again, this association was stronger among premenopausal women who had a family history of breast cancer. (*Journal of the National Cancer Institute*, March 17, 1999).

There is an exciting study underway right now at the AMC Cancer Research Center in Colorado with women who are at high risk for breast cancer. They are trying to find out if breast cancer risk is improved by eating more fruits and vegetables, and if eating 10 or more servings of produce a day is closer to the ideal amount. (You've heard of the "five a day" program? Well, that's based on the recommended *minimum* number of servings—five a day.)

They already have encouraging results to report. After just two weeks on the "10 or more servings of fruits and vegetables" diet, the women showed significantly lower levels of a certain type of cellular DNA damage thought to be associated with the development of cancer.

I know how hard I have to work at it to get my five servings of fruits and vegetables a day...so imagine how difficult it was to get these women to eat 10! These women showed us that it can be done. The women reported being in very good moods with lots of energy, never feeling better. But some women did say it was tedious preparing all the fruits and vegetables called for in the study recipes. In The Food Steps To Freedom (Chapter 4), we give you quick and painless was to get more fruits and vegetables...you won't have to lift a finger, or a recipe card.

Beans (lignins) and breast cancer

Lignins are phytoestrogens that have possible anticancer effects. They function as antioxidants: Preventing certain cellular changes that can lead to cancer. Women who eat lignin-rich foods are less likely to develop breast cancer than those with lower levels (*Harvard Health Letter*, March 1997).

You'll find lignins in certain fruits and vegetables, certain beans, seeds, and whole grains:

- **Fruits:** Pears, plums.
- **Vegetables:** asparagus, beets, bell peppers, broccoli, carrots, cauliflower, garlic, leeks, iceberg lettuce, onions, snow peas, squash, sweet potatoes, turnips, and the dried seaweeds (mekuba and hijiki).
- **Beans:** soybeans, lentils, navy beans, fava beans, pinto beans, and kidney beans.
- **Whole Grains:** wheat, oats, brown rice, corn, rye, barley, triticale, sorghum.
- **Oil Seeds:** flaxseed, rapeseeds (used to make canola oil), sunflower seeds, peanuts.

Flaxseed and breast cancer

Flaxseed contains great things, such as soluble fiber (helping you feel full sooner, gently keeping bowels moving, and lowering blood cholesterol); alphalinolenic acid (a plant form of omega-3 fatty acid which may also help reduce the risk of heart disease); and lignins. Trust me, you'll be hearing much about flaxseed in the future.

The lignin content of flaxseed is up to 800 times greater than that of other plant foods. University of Toronto researchers found that flaxseed reduced breast cancer growths in rats by more than 50 percent (*Flaxseed in Human Nutrition*, ADCS Press). We'll have to wait for results of human studies (which are now underway) to know if the cancer-fighting powers of flaxseed go beyond rats.

How much might be helpful to the general population? A moderate approach would be about a half tablespoon of ground flaxseed a few times a week.

Fat and breast cancer

There are actually three ways that fat might have something to do with breast cancer risk: the amount of fat on our bodies, the total amount of fat in our meals, and the type of fat in our meals. We don't know all the details yet, but it looks like we should do for cancer what we do for heart disease—strive to avoid eating meals high in saturated and animal fats.

Amount of fat

Some animal studies have demonstrated that tumor incidence goes up when more than 25 percent of the calories come from fat. Although population and animal studies have linked high fat consumption to increased breast cancer rates, some large controlled studies of women have failed to demonstrate the relationship. When many of the different studies on amount of fat and breast cancer risk were analyzed together, researchers concluded that reducing fat below 20 percent of total calories could reduce breast cancer risk (*Journal of the National Cancer Institute* 91:529, 1999).

How could the amount of fat influence breast cancer risk? One of the most promising explanations is that eating a lot less fat (less than 20 percent of calories) could result in eating fewer calories overall. Eating fewer calories may lead to less adipose tissue storage (lower body fat) and hormone production. Extra body fat around the middle is associated with higher levels of available estrogen and with increased breast cancer risk in postmenopausal women.

Another important thing to consider is this: When people work to lower the fat in their diet (if they are doing it the right way), they increase plant foods which increases vitamins, phytochemicals, and fiber (and may have a connection to lowering the breast cancer risk).

Everyone agrees we need larger, longer-term studies. The "Women's Health Initiative" (National Institutes of Health) started a study in 1994 with one group of participants eating less than 20 percent of total calories from fat. However, many studies demonstrated a weak association between breast cancer and the amount of fat we eat.

Eating only 20 percent of total calories from fat is fairly doable for motivated, produce-loving Americans. But much less than that is going to hurt—a lot. When you eat around 20 to 25 percent calories from fat you can still have some meat, some dairy, and some of your other favorite foods (There is still room for chocolate). Eating less than 10 percent of calories from fat spells the end of your previous eating habits as you have known them.

Types of fat

Saturated fat and trans fatty acids are the fats you want to watch. There has been a strong correlation between age-adjusted breast cancer death rates and animal fats (the more animal fat, the higher the death rates). This association only gets stronger as we pass menopause (*Medical Clinics of North America*, 77:725, 1993). When researchers analyzed 12 case-control studies of diet and breast cancer risk, they found two nutritional factors were linked to breast cancer risk: saturated fat in postmenopausal women increased it while high levels of vitamin C decreased it. This was probably due to higher amounts of fruits and vegetables in the diet (*Journal of the National Cancer Institute*, 82:561, 1990).

Eating foods with more omega-3 fatty acids than omega-6 fatty acids has been proven to inhibit the growth of breast cancer in rats. There is also evidence that omega-3 fatty acids can inhibit the growth of human breast cancer cells both in vitro (test tubes) and in explants (human tissue experiments) (*Eur J Cancer*, November 1998).

Fat on our bodies

Extra fat around the waist is linked to higher levels of estrogen production. In postmenopausal women, this in turn, appears to increase risk of breast cancer.

Fiber and breast cancer

In the early stages of breast cancer, some tumors are stimulated by excess amounts of estrogen circulating in the bloodstream. It is possible, therefore, that dietary factors that decrease circulating estrogen might help prevent breast tumor growth. One of the dietary factors is fiber, but not just any old type of fiber—wheat fiber. Some scientists believe fiber may hamper the growth of some early-stage breast tumors by binding with estrogen in the intestine, decreasing the amount of excess estrogen from being reabsorbed from the intestines and pumped into the bloodstream.

About 10 years ago, a review and analysis of 12 studies found a link between a high-fiber diet and a reduced risk of breast cancer. One even showed an association between increases in fiber and reductions in serum estrogen while the calories from fat remained unchanged (*American Journal of Clinical Nutrition*, 54:520, 1991). They found the fiber/estrogen association seemed to depend on the amount of fiber from wheat as well as how long the wheat fiber was supplemented.

I'm personally hoping there is a connection. Eating more fiber is something we should all be doing anyway—especially if we do it by eating more fruits, vegetables, and whole grains. Alas, another study came out that threw a wrench in the gears. Researchers analyzing data from the "Nurses' Health Study" concluded in 1992 that fiber intake has no influence on breast cancer risk in middle-aged women.

Fiber helps you eat less

Eating more fiber helps you eat less and perhaps even absorb fewer calories. It does this partly by lowering insulin levels circulating in our blood (insulin helps stimulate our appetite).

Fiber helps fill our stomach with bulk promoting a full feeling sooner. One study found that people ate smaller lunches after eating high-fiber breakfasts (*American Journal of Clinical Nutrition*, Dec. 1989). Some scientists suspect that fiber may speed up the time the food we eat spends in our intestine, possibly reducing the calories absorbed.

Alcohol and breast cancer

Although not considered definitive proof, a wide range of laboratory and population studies shows that alcohol can influence the initiation, promotion, and progression of cancer.

You might expect that high alcohol consumption has been linked to cancer of the liver, but it has also been linked to breast cancer as well as rectum, mouth, esophagus, pharynx, larynx, digestive tract, bladder, and lung cancers. And alcohol working with tobacco seems to have a greater chance of causing cancer than either does alone.

These are ways that alcohol may be linked to cancer:

- The alcohol is broken down in the body to a substance called acetaldehyde. Acetaldehyde has been found to have carcinogenic effects in laboratory studies.
- Alcohol may depress your immune system, impairing your body's ability to recognize and eliminate cancerous cells.
- Alcohol seems to decrease levels of vitamin A and E (two antioxidants that may play a role in preventing cancer).
- Women drinking about one ounce of pure alcohol (the amount in two average drinks) every day for three months were found to have higher levels of estrogen than were nondrinkers.
- There might be other ingredients in alcoholic beverages that could be associated with cancer formation (such as nitrosamines).

The Nurses' Health Study found that women who drank one or two drinks a day had a 50-percent higher rate of breast cancer than those who did not drink at all. Beer drinking seems to put men and women at higher risk than other alcoholic beverages.

Weight gain and breast cancer

Most of us women don't need any research to tell us that it is easier for women to become overweight then men—we already know. One reason for the difference between men and women concerning obesity may be that the fluctuations in reproductive hormone concentrations throughout women's lives predispose us to excess weight gain. But let's not spend time discussing *why* it is so easy for some women to gain weight through the years—let's talk about whether it increases the risk of breast cancer.

It may all come down to the fact that body fat produces estrogen. The theory is that weight gain raises the risk because the body fat produces estrogen, which may then prompt the growth of breast tumors. Harvard researchers noted, after tracking more than 95,000 nurses for 16 years, that 16 percent of all of the postmenopausal breast cancers could be traced to weight gain. There are several possible reasons for a link:

- Fatty tissues store carcinogenic chemicals.
- Taking in excessive calories may make it easier for cells to multiply.
- Fat stores may stimulate the production of extra estrogen (and high levels promote the growth of some breast tumors).

Chapter 4 has an entire section on what you can do about it, titled "What Are You 'Weight'ing For?" You can find it on page 73.

Soy, phytoestrogens, and breast cancer

One class of phytochemicals is phytoestrogens. Soy foods contain a type of phytoestrogen—isoflavones. Some studies suggest that soy isoflavones inhibit breast cancer development. The isoflavones are structurally similar to estrogens and researchers suspect the weak plant estrogen functions as an antiestrogen by competing with the more potent estrogen circulating in our bodies.

Some research suggests that a high intake of soy helps protect against breast cancer but this will be difficult to prove definitively. We can say that including soy foods changes your hormone levels and resulting in a longer menstrual cycle in premenopausal women (which is related to a lower risk of breast cancer).

Vitamin E food sources

Vitamin E can be found in good quantities in unprocessed whole grains. The milling and bleaching of wheat to make white flour takes most of the vitamin E out. Nuts, seeds (and the cooking oils they make), poultry, fish, and eggs all contribute vitamin E to the diet.

The bottom line

Epidemiological reports have been inconsistent. One researcher suggests that studies focusing on a single nutrient often fail to recognize potential interactions between nutrients (such as between fatty acids and antioxidant vitamins). The problem is that researchers most often study the effect of a specific nutrient on disease or risk. One British oncology researcher calls for studying the effect of a reduced fat intake paired with a diet rich in omega-3 fatty acids, vitamin E and retinoid, a combination he suspects will increase its effectiveness (*Eur J Cancer*, November 1998).

A good diet strengthens body defenses against environmental insults, whatever they may be. While the scientists sort out which compounds are carcinogenic, it makes sense to eat defensively. You'll find out what this means in Chapter 4.

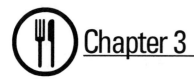 Chapter 3

Everything You Ever Wanted to Ask a Dietitian About Preventing Breast Cancer...

Q **Which cancers have the strongest associations with what you eat?**

Reducing risk through diet changes is thought to have the strongest associations with breast, colon/rectum, and prostate cancers (*Cancer*, 1998; 83:1425-32).

Q **What is it about soy that might make it helpful toward preventing breast cancer?**

Most of the interest in soy is based on studies that found that populations eating large amounts of soy have a much lower incidence of breast and prostate cancer (a four- to 10-fold lower incidence). Researchers have looked at the plant chemicals in soybeans to try to explain its positive health effects. They found that soybeans contain several classes of anticarcinogenic components: protease inhibitors (which may slow the rate of cancer division in cells), phytosterols (which seem to block estrogen), saponins (which may prevent cancer cells from multiplying), phenolic acids, phytic acid, and isoflavones. Isoflavones are similar in structure to a form of estrogen. Some researchers propose that the isoflavones (in premenopausal women) lower the amount of estrogen able to bind to receptor sites because isoflavones compete with estrogen. Soy has displayed anticarcinogenic activity in laboratory tests involving cancer of the breast (and prostate and colon cancers as well). And in some preliminary human trials, soy showed the potential to inhibit these cancers. The research on soy and breast cancer remains mixed so far, particularly for women who have or once had breast cancer. Most researchers agree that more work is needed before specific dietary recommendations can be made. In the meantime, it makes sense to include a variety of beans occasionally—including soy.

Q **What happens after menopause when you don't have high levels of estrogen circulating in your body? Do phytoestrogens, such as isoflavones, turn from *anti*estrogens to *pro*estrogens—stimulating the growth of estrogen-dependent cancers?**

This is a sticky subject and a question that continues to be investigated. Before menopause, plant estrogens, such as isoflavones, are thought to displace the more potent forms of estrogen in the body, discouraging the growth of estrogen-dependent cancers. But could the body confuse these plant estrogens as the more potent forms of estrogen that aren't made by the body after menopause, thus stimulating tumor growth? That's the big question. Some researchers think this isn't so much a concern if you are getting your isoflavones from food...but more of a concern if you are taking in isolated forms of isoflavones from supplements.

Let's go back to the beginning for a minute. In those studies of populations where soy is consumed in large amounts, do these women have a higher incidence of breast cancer after menopause? Two recent populations studies say no. One study found the risk of breast cancer decreased with increasing tofu intake in both pre- and postmenopausal women. Stay tuned for more information on soy and postmenopausal women—when the results of research going on right now become available.

Q **Are some soy foods better than others?**
Fermented soy products, such as soy sauce, have a different chemical composition than nonfermented soy. We don't yet know how this affects the potential anticarcinogenic properties of these products. Manufacturers and researchers are now publishing the isoflavone content of various soy-based products. But I think we can guess that it is probably better to get your soy serving from things like soy milk, tofu, tempeh, and miso rather than from soy flour, high-sodium soy sauce, or high-calorie soy oil. According to a USDA/Iowa State University Database on the Isoflavone Content of Foods, the following soy foods contain the highest amount isoflavones:

Soybeans, cooked or dry roasted are starting to be available in big supermarkets. I've even found canned organic soybeans. You can also buy soybeans frozen in pods. Cook them in their pod, then scoop out the soybeans inside for a different way to enjoy soybeans. Add soybeans to rice or casseroles or just eat them as a side dish. Dry roasted soybeans can be eaten out of your hand as a snack or add them as a topping to salads.

Tofu, the rubbery "cheese" from soy milk, takes on the flavor of whatever you cook it with. It comes in soft or firm textures. The soft (or silken) type of tofu can be pureed with things. The firm tofu is best diced into cubes or crumbled. A three-ounce slice contains about 50 calories.

Tempeh, the nutty-flavored soybean cake, has a firm texture and can be barbecued, crumbled into spaghetti sauce, or such. A three-ounce slice contains about 150 calories.

Soy milk is available in the dairy section of many supermarkets. The fresh soy milks (usually in cartons) taste the best by far. Soy milk can be used to make blender drinks, puddings, and in all types of baking and cooking.

Miso: You've heard of miso soup perhaps? Miso is a tasty salty paste and it adds zest to all kinds of things (sauces, soups, dressings, marinades, and so forth). It contains a fair amount of sodium though (about 600 mg per tablespoon).

Q **What about nitrosamines—are they something I should be worried about?**

In the 1970s scientists detected nitrosamines (known to be carcinogenic) in many favorite foods (cooked bacon and sausage, cured pork and dried beef, and so forth). Out of them all, bacon had one of the highest levels. Nitrosamines are formed during the breakdown of nitrites and nitrates, which are chemicals used to cure and preserve meats. Nitrates and nitrites are used because they give cured meats a pink look and protect against botulism (a potentially deadly bacteria). However there are a few different substances that actually help stop the formation of nitrosamines (from the nitrates and nitrites). For example, some meat-product manufacturers have been adding these substances to their wares:

- **Vitamins C and E (antioxidants).** On the label you won't see "vitamin C or E," you'll see their official names: ascorbic acid or ascorbate (vitamin C) or tocopherol (vitamin E).
- **P-coumaric and chlorogenic acids (found in fruits and vegetables).** If your favorite turkey bacon or reduced-fat hot dog doesn't have these good things added to it, add your own. Eat it with some fruits and vegetables high in vitamin C (citrus fruits and green vegetables).

Q **Does barbecuing contribute to cancer?**

Barbecuing and grilling have gotten bad reputations lately due to news that the yummy black char that forms when you grill or barbecue your food can contain carcinogenic substances. When you smoke or char meats, these substances, called Polycyclic Aromatic Hydrocarbons (PAHs), are deposited on the surface of the food. Much like nitrosamines, PAHs have been found to be carcinogenic. However, we should be even more concerned about HCAs (heterocyclic amines). HCAs, which can cause genetic mutations in cells, appear when high heat is applied to a combination of amino acids—primarily creatine (found in blood and muscle of animals). So far, we know HCAs cause tumors in animals and that they are most often associated with cancers of the gastrointestinal tract.

Some lab studies have suggested a connection between HCAs and breast tumors. HCAs are also suspected of working together with food fat to promote cancer growth. The latest scientific breakthrough with HCAs will have you hoping that caffeine keeps you up at night. The same enzyme that breaks down HCAs quickly to get rid of them also breaks down caffeine. Researchers have found that animals that break down HCAs quickly appear to be at greater risk for HCA-induced cancers, rather than the animals who break them down slowly (slow metabolizers). In a recent study with female rats, more breast cancer was seen in the fast metabolizers than in the slow (Madhu Purewal, Ph.D., M.D., Anderson Cancer Center in Houston, Texas).

How can you know if you qualify as a "fast metabolizer"? If you can drink a caffeinated beverage (such as regular coffee, tea, or cola) at 8:30 p.m. and still get a good night's sleep, you are considered to be a "fast" metabolizer. It might be extra important that HCAs not be a regular guest at your dinner table.

So what do you do? Don't toss the grill just yet. There are a few things you can do to help safeguard your grilled food:

1. Choose marinades that are low in oil to minimize fat dripping onto the coals and causing high flames.
2. Trim visible fat from meat before marinating and grilling.
3. Eat your grilled meat with fruits and vegetables rich in vitamin C and beta carotene.
4. Precook meat for a few minutes in a microwave oven before putting it on the grill. Not only does this cut

down on the time the meat is on the grill, but it removes juices, reducing the amount of HCAs that can be produced.

5. Don't barbecue every day—keep it as an occasional treat.
6. Don't overcook your meat. Generally, the more well done the meat, the more HCAs it contains.

Q Are HCAs also found in fish and poultry, blackened dishes, burnt toast or grilled vegetables?

Bread and vegetables do not have the amounts of amino acids and creatine needed to form HCAs. However, fish and poultry do. Remember the HCAs form when cooked at high temperatures. Blackened dishes do obviously "blacken," but usually due to the charring of a breaded coating, not the actual meat. These would not be significant sources of HCAs.

Q What are your recommendations for vitamin or mineral supplements for fairly healthy women?

The science behind supplements and health is still being figured out with new information and research surfacing all the time. Based on what we know so far, I can make a few common-sense supplement suggestions. These are things I would tell anyone interested in being as healthy as they can be or anyone interested in improving their odds with chronic disease. The RDA (recommended daily allowance) represents the basic levels that satisfy the nutritional needs of healthy people. Most Americans fall short on meeting the RDA for most of the nutrients on a daily basis.

Another thing to consider is that the RDA wasn't designed to help fend off chronic disease. Some researchers suggest that taking certain vitamin or minerals above the RDA amounts may *help* in reducing the risk of several age-related illnesses. The supplements that have come up in research thus far are vitamins E and C, selenium, and the carotenoids (a phytochemical family of which beta carotene is a member).

So what can you do? You put your best foot forward—which is—and always will be—food. You want to get these important nutrients and phytochemicals from food. In food they are balanced, they are in naturally occurring amounts, and they compliment the nutrients and phytochemicals that we may have not discovered yet. Beyond this, it is a good idea for most of us to take a complete and balanced vitamin/mineral supplement and perhaps consider 200 to 400 IU (international units) of vitamin E (or mixed tocopherols). This is the amount that proves to be beneficial in research. However, it is very difficult to take in more than 30 IU of vitamin E from food alone. As with any nutritional supplements, you'll want to run your plan by your doctor, nurse practitioner, or pharmacist before going forward. You'll want to make sure it won't interfere with any medications you are taking.

Q **I know I should be eating more produce, but should I be concerned about pesticide residues and cancer risk?**

Fewer than 1 percent of all cancers are attributed to pesticides and other manufactured chemicals in air, water, soil, and food. Compare that with the estimated 60 to 70 percent of all cancers linked to lifestyle factors you can control. Don't get me wrong, it is still a good idea to wash all produce thoroughly in water, scrubbing the skin, removing outer leaves, and so forth. This not only reduces pesticide residues but also gets rid of dirt or bacteria that could make you sick. I generally try to buy seasonal produce and not rely too heavily on imported grapes and other fruits coming from countries with lax food safety and pesticide regulations.

I was surprised to read in a report from Consumers Union (*Consumer Reports*, March 1999) that according to their findings, more pesticide residues were found on domestic produce than on imports—except for imported grapes, tomatoes, and carrots. Recently a panel of experts from the United States and Canada reviewed more than 50 studies and concluded the benefits of eating fruits and vegetables far outweigh the potential risks from pesticides.

That doesn't mean we shouldn't try to use less pesticides. What pesticides do to the human body is not entirely known. Perhaps more importantly, we know little about how they might interact with each other. This could be a reason that you see more and more organic produce available. You may wonder which fruits and vegetables would we reap the biggest benefits from buying organic, and which are more pesticide-prone. Two reports came out in 1999, One from the Environmental Working Group, a nonprofit consumer organization, and one from the Consumer Union. Their rankings of fruits and vegetables with the highest pesticide residues didn't exactly agree with each other but between the two of them you can come up with a loose list of produce that you might want to buy organic when available and affordable. The Consumer Union (*Consumer Reports*, March 1999) and the Environmental Working Group (February 1999) found the following as having the highest pesticide residues: apples, spinach, peaches, pears, grapes, celery, and green beans. (Consumers Union listed tomatoes, lettuce, and carrots as having a "dishonorable" mention, whereas the

---

F.Y.I.   **How to cut pesticide risk at home**

- Buy organic versions of the more pesticide-prone produce listed above when available and affordable.
- Thoroughly wash fruits and vegetables with cool, running water, scrubbing to remove surface when needed.
- Throw away the outer leaves of lettuce and greens, where pesticide residues tend to be higher.
- Peel the pesticide-prone produce items, especially when serving them to children.

Environmental Working Group didn't list them in their "terrible 10." The Environmental Working Group listed strawberries and potatoes in their "terrible 10," where Consumers Union didn't list them in their "hit list.")

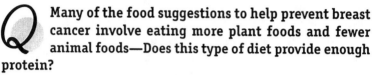 **Many of the food suggestions to help prevent breast cancer involve eating more plant foods and fewer animal foods—Does this type of diet provide enough protein?**

In America, protein tends to be overrated. First of all, most Americans get more than two times the protein they actually need. Too much protein may even be linked to a variety of health problems. Scientists used to think you needed to eat plant protein which complemented the animal-based proteins in the same meal (to make "complete" proteins). We now know this "complementing" takes place over many hours. By eating a variety of plant-based foods every day you will get the "building blocks" (essential amino acids) you need for growth and good health.

Do you have another question?

Do you have a question on diet and breast cancer that wasn't answered here? There are a few great places you can go with your questions. You'll find the list at the end of Chapter 1 (pages 20-21).

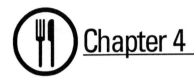 ## Chapter 4

The 10 Food Steps to Freedom

C ancer takes hold in many ways, most of them not yet fully understood, and what works for one individual may not work as well for the next. We are miles away from any guaranteed protection against breast cancer. But at this point, we are looking at improving our odds against the cancer by including (or avoiding) certain foods and nutrients in our diet.

In addition to suggesting foods that might help you, the Food Steps below may offer some protection by giving you a list of things to avoid. However, if you had to choose which to focus on, choose eating more of the foods that might help protect you against cancer. Why? The most important effects of diet seem to be through *inhibiting* the cancer process (*Food, Nutrition, and the Prevention of Cancer: a global perspective*, 1997, American Institute of Cancer Research).

The report cited above was groundbreaking because in it, scientists, after looking at the available research, made some conclusions that we can all benefit from. They found it was:

- "Probable" that vegetables and fruit decreased risk of breast cancer.
- "Possible" that carotenoids in foods decrease breast cancer risk.
- "Possible" that fiber decreases breast cancer risk.
- "Possible" that physical activity decreases breast cancer risk.

(You will find all of these represented in the 10 Food Steps to Freedom.)

Which foods/food components might increase risk? The report concluded that it was:

- "Probable" that alcohol increases risk of breast cancer.
- "Possible" that meat increases the risk of breast cancer.
- "Possible" that both total fat and saturated and animal fat increases breast cancer risk.
- "Probable" that obesity increases the risk of breast cancer.

(You will find all of these represented in the 10 Food Steps to Freedom as well.)

When looking at the following 10 Food Steps to Freedom, you can't help but notice that many of the steps are moving us gently toward a more plant-based diet. You can look at this two ways: Eating fewer animal foods or eating more plant foods. Both are probably best. Please realize that I'm not suggesting that we eliminate animal foods—I'm just suggesting that we, as Americans, will probably be better served with smaller portions of meats and taking every opportunity to add plant foods.

Food Steps 1 and 2: Enjoy more fruits and enjoy more vegetables

Why am I splitting up fruits and vegetables and giving each their own food step? Well, because they each deserve star billing—that's how important they are. Fruits and vegetables are important in a defensive eating plan. Fruits contribute some nutrients and phytochemicals, while vegetables offer others. They have many protective substances in common as well. There are powerful antioxidants in both and they both boast a variety of fiber. For a list of fruits and vegetables bursting in antioxidants, carotenoids, and other important phytochemicals, see "The most powerful produce" in Chapter 7 (page 139).

In more than 100 research studies, people who ate a lot of fruits and vegetables were only about half as likely to develop cancer as those who rarely ate those foods. Some people just take supplements without eating fruits or vegetables. The problem with that is, the benefits may be from something in fruits and vegetables that hasn't been isolated yet. Or the most benefit could come from the way the various nutrients interact with each other. So do yourself a favor—just eat the fruits and vegetables and skip most of those fancy supplements.

How many fruits and vegetables?

I always try to avoid reinventing the wheel so I'll use *The Dietary Guidelines for Americans* (U.S. Department of Agriculture and U.S. Department of Health and Human Services), which suggests two to four servings of fruit and three to five servings of vegetables per day. The number of servings should increase based on your need for energy. The "five-a-day" program you may have heard about (teaching people that they need a minimum of five servings of fruits and vegetables a day) takes the minimum number for each of these food groups and adds them together. However, when it comes to breast cancer prevention, let's take the higher number given and add them together: four servings of fruit and five servings of vegetables a day.

I'll admit that this is hard to do. But it is a great eating habit to aspire to. One thing I've noticed is as I strive to fit these nine servings a day I can't help but eat less of certain foods that aren't doing as much for me in terms of nutrition.

10 sure-proof ways to do it

Most of us are already well aware we should be eating more fruits and vegetables. But knowing and doing are two separate things. Well, why aren't we doing it? Some people say it is because they aren't as convenient as snack foods and fast food. Others say they simply aren't in the habit. I think we would all eat more fruits and vegetables if we just had our mothers prepare them—someone to take the time to turn them into fun fruit salads or colorful green salads, snack trays, tasty side dishes, or inventive entrées. This takes time, talent, and lots of love. Here are some ways we can "mother" ourselves into getting more fruits and vegetables:

1. Pack your desk or car with your favorite dried fruits— they will keep for weeks.
2. Buy baby carrots and celery sticks and put them out before dinner with an easy-to-make dip (mix some Ranch dip mix with a light or fat-free sour cream).
3. Take time Sunday or at the beginning or end of the work week to make a large spinach salad or a veg-etable-fortified lettuce salad, and store it (without dressing) in an airtight container. A crisp salad with lunch or dinner is only a few seconds away for the next few days.
4. Every few days make a point of going to your super-market and picking out the best-tasting and freshest in-season fruits. But the fruit doesn't do anyone any good sitting in the fruit bowl or crisper—You've got to remember to serve it. Put it out as a snack for the family. Add a few slices or wedges of fruit to each lunch or dinner plate.
5. With a few chops of a knife, you can turn a few pieces of fruit into a gorgeous fruit salad. Drizzle lemon, pineapple, or orange juice over the top and toss to coat (the vitamin C helps prevent browning).
6. Buy your favorite fruits in the winter—just buy them frozen or canned in juice or light syrup.

7. Stock your refrigerator at work and home with your favorite fruit juices (make sure they are 100-percent fruit juice). You can often buy them in individual servings so you can grab them as you are running out the door.
8. Make a point to include a vegetable with your lunch.
9. Make sure to eat vegetables when you go out for a meal at a restaurant or deli.
10. Enjoy fruit as a dessert or add fruit to your dessert when possible. For specific ideas, see "Shopping with a sweet tooth" in Chapter 7 (page 130).

The great salad experiment

What do most people order in a restaurant to compliment their lunch or dinner entrée? A green salad, of course! When you go to a party, a potluck, or a restaurant do you find yourself oohing and aahing over the beautiful fresh fruit or green salads? I know *I* do!

One day as I was staring at an empty fruit salad bowl that I filled just the day before, I formed my salad hypothesis:

If people had already-prepared, wonderfully fresh fruit and green salads available in their refrigerator, where all they had to do was grab a bowl and fork, they would find themselves miraculously eating more fruit and vegetables than they ever thought possible.

In order to do this you'll need a little pep talk regarding the amount of extra time this salad making requires. It requires investment of about 10 minutes every few days. You rinse, chop and toss just once to have glorious salad available for several days.

Some salad suggestions

I try and assemble my salads right after I get home from the supermarket. When you are unpacking your groceries, just put the fruit and vegetables on the counter until you get a moment to rinse, chop, and toss. I find that once the fruits and vegetables reach the crisper drawer, there's only a 50 percent chance they're ever going to make it out again.

If I can't get to the fruits and vegetables shortly after I bring them home from the supermarket, then I wait until both my children (and sometimes my husband) have gone to bed. When the house is quiet and no one is pulling on my apron strings, I position my cutting board along with all my fruits and vegetables in front of the TV and I chop and peel to whatever TV show suits my fancy.

Do potatoes count?

At least one cancer research agency is suggesting potatoes don't count toward your grand total of fruits and vegetables. Could this be because in this country more than half of every potato eaten is a French fry? Potatoes do contribute vitamin C, fiber, and other nutrients and make some of our favorite side dishes. It's just that compared to the French fry, you are definitely better off filling your plate with nutrient-packed vegetables (such as broccoli, spinach, cauliflower, and carrots).

Food Step 3: Work a carotenoid-rich food into your day

It is "possible" that carotenoids (a family of phytochemicals) in food decrease the risk of breast cancer. So far that's all we have to go on. But when I suggest you work a carotenoid-rich food into your day, I'm asking you to eat more of certain fruits and vegetables—fruits and vegetables that also happen to have all sorts of other nutritional attributes going for them as well.

Most people have heard of the most famous member of the carotenoid family: beta carotene. But there are actually many other carotenes being studied. It looks like part of the power of the carotenes comes in their working together. That's why eating a food rich in many of the carotenes is probably going to benefit your body more than taking a pill with only beta carotene. (For a list of carotenoid-rich foods see the section "The most powerful produce" in Chapter 7 [page 139].)

Cruciferous (cabbage family) vegetables also seem to offer potential cancer fighting benefits. There is a phytochemical found in cruciferous family vegetables known as indole-3-carbinol that acts as an active chemopreventive and an antiestrogen. Can they help prevent breast cancer? It's an idea that has some potential. Studies have linked indoles to cervical and prostate cancer risk reduction. In studies with mice, researchers found that indole-3-carbinol could be useful to prevent cervical cancer. Other researchers believe it may be an effective chemopreventive or therapeutic agent against prostate cancer by inhibiting the growth of prostate cancer cells and by protecting cells from oxidative stress.

Citrus fruits, as most people already know, are brimming with the antioxidant vitamin C. By many cancer researchers, vitamin C is thought to be the most versatile cancer-fighting antioxidant. After examining 90 epidemiological studies, one researcher reported "strong" evidence for vitamin C-having protective effects on the esophagus, oral cavity, stomach, and pancreas along with "somewhat strong" evidence for its protecting against cervical, breast, and rectal cancers.

And there is more to citrus than just vitamin C. Citrus fruits also contain powerful phytochemicals (flavonoids, limonoids, and cumarins) that chemically inhibit induced cancer in animal studies. One recent study found that feeding a citrus product (double strength orange juice) delayed the onset of breast cancer in rats (*Nutr Cancer*, 1996, 26: 167). There is much more we need to know regarding citrus and breast cancer, but this just is one more reason to pick up an orange or grapefruit.

Calling all antioxidants

Oxygen damage to your cells is partly responsible for the effects of aging and chronic disease. Because oxidation is harmful, it makes sense that antioxidants would be beneficial. You can help your body fight free radicals by:

1. Limiting your exposure to the external hazards. Wear sunscreen, stop smoking and avoid secondhand smoke. Drink alcohol in moderation.

2. Consuming foods rich in antioxidants. Antioxidants protect us by donating electrons to stabilize and neutralize the harmful effect of free radicals. But different antioxidants have different jobs so it's important to get all of them. Some deactivate free radicals; others transform them to less toxic compounds. These antioxidants include beta carotene, vitamin A, vitamin C, vitamin E, and selenium. Selenium is part of an enzyme that functions as an antioxidant (see more on selenium in Food Step 4).

If you ate these 3 foods every day...

Ever since Chapter 2 you've been reading about the possible anticancer activities of the cruciferous vegetables, antioxidants, and phytochemicals like the carotene family. Many people just want me to tell them which foods to eat almost every day. If I told you to eat certain fruits and vegetables every day, you would probably grow to loathe them (if you didn't hate them already). And remember that variety is always important for health of the body as well as the mind.

Having said that, let's just suppose you won't tire of eating a few popular nutrient-packed produce items on most days. What would happen nutritionally if you ate some broccoli (or spinach), a glass of calcium-fortified orange juice, and a carrot? There are about 20 carotenoids in an orange that have significant antioxidant activity and the more than 60 flavonoids in citrus possess a wide range of properties including strong antioxidant activity. The table on the facing page shows a sample of what each of these will contribute to your day's nutrition total:

Just a few of the vitamins & minerals you'll get

1 cup broccoli (or 2 cups fresh chopped spinach)	• Antioxidant vitamins C and E • Beta carotene and other carotenoids • Cruciferous vegetable; contains indole-3 carbinol • Other nutrients such as folic acid • Phytochemicals such as the flavonoids and phytoestrogens • Five grams of fiber
8 ounces of calcium-fortified orange juice(with pulp)	• Carotenoids (phytochemicals) • Antioxidant vitamin C • The antioxidant-like vitamin, folic acid • Flavonoids (antioxidant phytochemicals) • Pectin (soluble fiber)
1 cup cooked carrots	• Beta carotene and other carotenoids • Phytoestrogens and other phytochemicals • Folic acid and other important vitamins • Five grams of fiber

Go for the garlic and onions

Garlic and onions may not technically be the kind of vegetables you serve as a side dish with dinner but they have the powerful phytochemicals of a super vegetable. Animal studies have shown that garlic and the allyl sulfur compounds it contains (onions also contain them) inhibit different stages of the carcinogenic process potentially effecting the colon, lung, skin, and breast. Recently, it was found that garlic compounds blocked the action of certain oxidizing enzymes that activate carcinogens.

A French study (*Eur J Epidemiol*, 1998, Dec;14[8]: 737) found breast cancer risk decreased as cereal fiber and garlic and onions increased. More needs to be known on this but recent research gives us a good start. Go forth and enjoy your garlic and onions—they do seem to be one of those foods that can help lower cancer risk.

Food Step 4: Eat more fiber, especially from wheat

Fiber has been known as a good thing for years now. Different fiber sources, however, have gotten more publicity than others from time to time. Wheat bran and wheat germ had their day in the 1970s, where oat bran ruled the fiber roost in the 90s. We are hopefully going to be more informed about fiber in the new century. We now know that there isn't any one type of fiber food that is "the answer" to all our health woes. A variety of fiber is in order, with each type of fiber benefiting our bodies in different ways.

For example, oat bran and other soluble fiber have cholesterol lowering and blood sugar lowering effects. Wheat fiber and other insoluble fiber (fiber that doesn't mix with water) is better known for its link in helping prevent constipation, colon cancer and now possibly breast cancer.

Women who ate a daily half-cup serving of All-Bran (worth 10 grams of fiber) saw drops in their estrogen levels. If high levels of estrogen stimulate breast cancer (as some experts think), eating more dietary fiber could end up being very helpful in breast cancer prevention (*Nutrition*, June 1997). Whole grains offer a wide range of nutrients and phytochemicals that may work together to optimize health and help prevent disease—possibly even breast cancer. Phytochemicals found in whole grains (protease inhibitors, phytic acid, phenolics and saponins) have all been found to reduce risk of breast and colon cancers in animal studies (*Nutrition Updates*, Fall 1999).

Whole wheat is giving us much more than just grams of fiber—whole wheat is rich in antioxidants too. The bran portion of the wheat, in addition to the fiber, offers us B vitamins, minerals, and scores of phytochemicals (lignans, phytoestrogens, phenolic acids, phytate, and plant sterols). The germ of the wheat is rich in oil (most of which is unsaturated), vitamin E, and phytochemicals (such as plant sterols). A USDA researcher reports on some studies that have determined that one serving of whole grain breakfast cereal provides antioxidants equal to the amount in a day's supply of fruits and vegetables.

You won't believe all the ways that fiber helps our bodies. What strikes me most about fiber is that there is both a short-term and long-term health payoff. Fiber helps us feel better and fight disease...both now and later. Here is the short list of benefits:

- Fiber holds onto water and ends up softening stools in the large intestine, which helps prevent constipation. Preventing constipation can then help the body prevent hemorrhoids, varicose veins, hiatus hernia, and diverticulosis.
- Fiber speeds the passage of food through the intestines and can reduce the amount of calories your body is able to absorb. It may also reduce the time that intestinal tissue is exposed to cancer-causing agents in the food.
- Some forms of soluble fiber can also help lower blood cholesterol levels, either by binding to certain lipids (such as cholesterol), carrying it out of the body via the stools, or by other possible mechanisms.
- High-fiber foods, because of fiber's ability to hold onto water in the stomach and intestines, gives us a feeling of fullness and satisfaction after a meal. This can help some of us eat less at each meal.

- In general, high-fiber foods are often high in nutrients and low in fat and calories.

So how much fiber are we talking about?

We Americans don't do a good job of meeting the fiber recommendations. The average U.S. diet contains less than half of the recommended amount. (The National Cancer Institute recommends 20 to 30 grams per day.) When discussing fiber recommendations, women will often say to me, "I have whole wheat toast in the morning!" Then I usually say, "Okay, so where are you getting the remaining 26 grams?" Don't get me wrong, enjoying whole wheat or whole grain toast is terrific, but don't think that's the end to your fiber needs for the day.

To meet the fiber recommendations, women have to pull out all the stops. Switching to whole grain products and foods when possible is a great place to start. To get 20 to 30 grams of fiber a day you need to make fruits and vegetables a part of almost every meal. You need to have a few fiber tricks up your sleeve—namely eating legumes (peas and beans) as well as concentrated fiber foods (brans and high fiber cereals with bran, psyllium seed, and so forth). Some people feel comfortable using the fiber supplements available at the pharmacy, but you really need to consult your doctor or practitioner before using these products. Some of them contain chemicals (intestinal stimulants) that act as a laxative in the body—steer clear of those.

Where do you find fiber?

Find a plant food and you find fiber. This means fruits, vegetables, whole grains and whole-grain products, and legumes. Take a peek below to see which foods have about three grams of fiber or more per serving. Of course, the amount of calories and fiber can vary by brands, but this will give you the basic information for most foods. (You'll find more information on food products containing fiber in Chapter 7.)

Fiber in your favorite foods

Food	Calories	Fiber (g)
Breads		
Whole wheat bagel, 1	145	5.5
Oat bran bagel, 1	173	7.5
Pita pocket, whole wheat, 1	120	3.2
Whole wheat bread, 2 slices	172	4.4
Mixed grain or whole wheat English muffin, 1	102	4.8
Oat bran muffin, 2 5/8-inches	130	3.5
Wheat bran muffin made with 2 percent milk, 1	160	4
Cookies & Snacks		
Fig Newton, Nabisco, 4	214	3.6
Popcorn, plain, 3 cups	92	3.6
Fruits		
Apple slices with peel, 1 1/2 cups	98	3.1
Apple rings (dried), 10	156	5.5
Apricot halves, 1 cup	74	3
Apricot halves (dried), 1/3 cup	103	3.3
Banana slices, 1 cup	138	3
Blackberries or boysenberries, 1 cup	75	6.3
Dates, 5	114	3.1
Figs, 2	74	3.2
Grapefruit sections, 1 cup	74	3
Mango slices, 1 cup	107	4.5
Orange sections, 1 cup	85	3.4
Peach slices, 1 cup	73	3
Pear (Bartlett), 1	98	4
Plum slices, 1 cup	90	3.2
Prunes, 5	100	4
Raspberries, 1 cup	60	4.9
Strawberries, 1 1/2 cups whole	64	3.3

Fiber in your favorite foods, continued

Food	Calories	Fiber (g)
Grains & Pasta		
Barley, pearled, cooked, 1 cup	193	7.8
Barley, whole, cooked, 1 cup	270	13.6
Kasha, cooked, 1/2 cup	343	9.4
Oat bran, dry, 1/4 cup	58	3.7
Oats, rolled, dry, 1/2 cup	156	4.2
Rice, brown, long grain, cooked, 1 cup	217	3.5
Spinach egg noodles, cooked, 1 cup	211	3.7
Wheat bran, crude, 1/4 cup	32	6.3
Whole wheat flour, 1/4 cup	102	3.5
Whole wheat macaroni, cooked, 1 cup	174	5.2
Whole wheat spaghetti, cooked, 1 cup	174	6.3

Hot Cereal (cold cereal is listed in Chapter 7)

Food	Calories	Fiber (g)
Corn grits, cooked, 1 cup	145	4.5
Maypo, 3/4 cup	128	4.2
Oatmeal, instant, 1 packet maple and brown sugar flavor	163	3.3
Ralston, 1 cup	253	6
Wheatena, 1 cup	136	6.5

Nuts & Seeds

Food	Calories	Fiber (g)
Almonds, 1/4 cup dry roasted	202	3.5
Pistachio, 1/4 cup dry roasted	185	3.5
Pumpkin seeds, dry roasted, 1/4 cup	186	4.8
Soy nut/soybean, dry roasted, 1/4 cup	193	3.5

Vegetables

Food	Calories	Fiber (g)
Artichoke hearts, frozen, boiled, 4.5 oz.	54	6.3
Asparagus, cooked, 1 cup	45	4
Blackeyed peas, boiled, 1/2 cup	112	7.3
Bok choy, cooked, 1 cup	20	3
Broccoli, raw, 1 cup	18	3

Fiber in your favorite foods, continued

Food	Calories	Fiber (g)
Vegetables, continued		
Broccoli, steamed, 1 cup	44	4.7
Brussels sprouts, cooked, 1 cup	61	7.2
Cabbage, savoy, cooked, 1 cup	35	4
Carrots, baby, raw, 10 each	38	3.2
Carrots, cooked, 1 cup	70	5
Cauliflower, steamed, 1 cup	31	3
Corn, white, boiled, 1/2 cup	88	4.7
Green beans, cooked, 1 cup	44	4
Greens (beet), boiled, 1 cup	39	4.2
Greens (dandelion), boiled, 1 cup	35	3
Greens (mustard), boiled, 1 cup	21	3
Greens (turnip), boiled, 1 cup	29	4.4
Hominy, cooked, 1 cup	145	9.4
Kohlrabi, boiled, 1 cup	48	3.2
Parsnip, boiled, 1 cup	126	7
Peas, green, boiled, 1/2 cup	62	4.4
Potato, baked with skin, 1 cup	133	3
Potato, mashed w/ whole milk, 1 cup	162	4.2
Potato fries (Ore Ida Golden Crinkles), 5 ounces	204	3.4
Pumpkin, canned, 1/2 cup	42	3.4
Rutabaga cubes, boiled, 1 cup	66	3
Snow peas (pea pods), boiled, 1 cup	67	4.5
Spinach, raw, 2 cups	24	3
Spinach, boiled from frozen, 1 cup	53	5
Squash (acorn), baked cubes, 1 cup	115	9
Squash (butternut), baked cubes, 1 cup	82	6
Squash (hubbard) baked, 1 cup	120	6.4
Sweet potatoes, mashed, 1/2 cup	103	3
Swiss chard, boiled, 1 cup	35	3.7
Tomatoes, canned, 1 cup	48	4.3
Tomato sauce, 1 cup	74	3.4

Fiber in your favorite foods, continued

Food	Calories	Fiber (g)
Vegetables, continued		
Turnips, boiled/mashed, 1 cup	42	4.6
Yams, boiled/baked, 1 cup	158	5.3
Beans		
Adzuki, cooked, 1/2 cup	147	6
Black, cooked, 1/2 cup	114	7.5
Fava, cooked, 1/2 cup	94	4.3
Garbanzo, cooked, 1/2 cup	134	4
Great Northern, canned, 1 cup	148	7
Kidney, canned, 1/2 cup	109	8.2
Lentil, boiled from dry, 1 cup	230	9
Lima, baby, boiled, 1/2 cup	94.5	6
Navy, canned, 1/2 cup	148	7
Pinto, canned, 1/2 cup	94	4.2
Pinto, refried, canned, 1/2 cup	135	13.4
Soybeans, boiled from dry, 1/2 cup	149	5.4
White, canned, 1/2 cup	153	6.3

5 steps to fiber

1. **Switch to "whole" grains when you can** (such as brown or wild rice, whole wheat or whole grain breads, whole wheat tortillas).

2. **Cook with whole-wheat flour more often.** I use half or one-third whole-wheat flour and the rest unbleached white flour when making breads, muffins, or pizza at home. If you use all whole wheat you might not be happy with the results. But using a third or half seems to work out well most of the time.

3. **Reach for a whole grain breakfast hot or cold cereal when you can.** (For a list of cereals with 5 grams or more of fiber, see "Fiber first thing in the morning" in Chapter 7 [page 129].)

4. **Get plenty of fruits and vegetables.** Add fruit in the morning, fruit as a snack, and fruit as or with dessert. Include a vegetable with lunch, vegetable sticks as a snack or pre-dinner munchie, and enjoy a couple vegetables with dinner.

5. **Break down the barrier to beans.** Eating beans comes more naturally to other cultures and countries across the globe. Enjoying popular foods from other countries, such as those from Mexico, can bring you closer to beans. Here are some other ways to boost your bean intake:

- Add beans to soups, stews, or chili that you normally make at home.

- Buy the better-tasting canned bean soups or vegetarian chili to have around at home for a quick side dish or snack.

- Make a quick three-bean salad by just tossing a light dressing with three different types of canned beans. (see recipe in Chapter 6).

- Sprinkle some beans on a green salad, pasta salad, Southwestern chicken salad, or taco salad.

- Make a delicious bean dip for parties. When the party is over, keep it in the refrigerator for a quick snack.

- If you are ordering a chicken or beef burrito in a restaurant or burrito bar, ask that they add whole pinto beans to the burrito for an easy fiber boost.

There's more to beans than fiber

Beans are a nutritionally efficient food because they have so many health benefits in one little package:

- They appear to slow the absorption of glucose in the bloodstream, thus curbing your appetite longer.

- They are packed full of fiber.

- They can contain phytoestrogens (soybeans contains isoflavones, while lentils, soybeans, kidney beans, navy beans, pinto and fava beans are rich in lignins— another kind of phytoestrogen).
- Beans contain other beneficial phytochemicals that help protect the body from disease, including protease inhibitors, phytosterols, and saponins.
- They are a low-fat source of plant protein.
- They are great sources of many vitamins and minerals we need more of as we age, such as folic acid and vitamin B-6.
- A diet rich in bean fiber tends to significantly decrease total blood cholesterol and produce a better HDL (good) cholesterol to LDL (bad) cholesterol ratio.

But beans give you gas...

Try adding beans slowly to your diet. Start by eating about a half cup of beans two times a week. Use canned beans and rinse them well before adding them to your recipes. And try over-the-counter gas fighting remedies, such as Beano, if you continue to have a problem. Beano contains enzymes that break down the gas-producing sugars in beans.

But beans take too much time to soak...

Don't soak them—use canned beans instead. How hard can opening a can be? Just dump the beans in a colander and rinse. You can find all types of canned beans today—even pinto and soybeans in some supermarkets.

Beans and selenium

Why is selenium important in a book about breast cancer? Selenium is an important mineral that is an important part of a number of enzymes that act as antioxidants.

Recently, studies have been suggesting that selenium might protect against cancer (including possibly breast cancer). A study on mice found that mice receiving a special high-selenium soybean meal had significantly less tumors after being induced with cancer cells than mice on a low-selenium soy meal (Creighton University School of Medicine, Omaha, Ne.). Recent clinical studies suggest that supplemental selenium (at safe levels) can also reduce cancer risk for humans (Gerald Combs Jr., Ph.D., Division of Nutritional Sciences, Cornell University). Apparently the effective dose of selenium can be easily had by eating a good diet.

As with many minerals, selenium is toxic at very high levels. Whatever excess amounts of selenium we take in collects in our body tissues. So the trick to selenium is getting enough without getting too much. The best way to do this is to get most of your selenium from food, staying away from selenium supplements. Remember, if you are taking a complete vitamin mineral supplement (such as Centrum), you are already getting the RDA for selenium (55 mcg [micrograms] is the RDA for adult women). Along with eating beans fairly frequently and whole grains as often as possible, you will have your selenium bases covered.

Whole grains, legumes, and Brazil nuts are the best plant sources of selenium (most fruits and vegetables contain only small amounts but some are rather potent). Selenium is also found in seafood, meats, and eggs. Here are some suggestions to increase your plant-food supply of selenium:

- Making a sandwich with whole wheat bread (or a whole-wheat English muffin or bagel) gets you one-third of the way to the RDA (20 mcg).
- A bowl of oatmeal or whole grain breakfast cereal contributes about 10 mcg.
- A cup of whole wheat pasta adds up to 40 mcg.
- A cup of brown rice brings you about 20 mcg (but white rice isn't far behind—15 mcg per cup).
- Dried Brazil nuts are almost like selenium supplements. One tablespoon already contains 250 mcg.

- A half cup of canned beans is worth about 3to 8 mcg. (A cup of black-eyed peas gives you five mcg.)
- One cup of boiled Brussels sprouts contributes 21 mcg.
- A half cup of cucumber slices (with peel) contains 6 lmcg.
- Five mushrooms have 11 mcg.

Tofu or not tofu, that is the question

It's no surprise that tofu contains some fiber and is loaded with phytoestrogens and other phytochemicals that are found in most soy foods. One of the phytoestrogens in tofu and soy that researchers are particularly interested in studying is isoflavone.

When nine studies on soy's relationship with breast cancer were analyzed, a high soy intake was associated with a modest statistically significant reduction in risk in premenopausal women. Researchers found no protective effect at all in postmenopausal women. Some studies have even suggested potentially adverse effects of soy. However, starting in early 1999, isoflavone extract from soy is being used in phase I prevention trials for breast and prostate cancer by the National Cancer Institute.

In the meantime, you might consider some soy foods especially if they seem to bring you relief from hot flashes during perimenopause. Besides that, there is probably nothing wrong with enjoying a nice soy meal every now and then (especially if it is replacing a high animal-fat entrée).

How much isoflavone might be needed to have an effect in women? Researchers are still figuring this out but is appears to be around 30 mg/day, the amount in about:

- 2 1/2 ounces of tofu.
- 2 1/2 ounces of tempeh.
- 2 1/2 ounces of miso.
- 50 grams (1 3/4 ounces) miso soup mix (dry).
- 8 ounces of soy milk.
- 15 grams of dry roasted soybeans.
- 100 grams (3.5 ounces) soy paste.

If you are new to the fiber scene...

Take it slow. Most people's bodies adjust to eating more fiber within about six weeks. While your body is "adjusting" you may notice gas, diarrhea, and abdominal pain. Increase your fiber slowly and drink plenty of water and you will hopefully scare away these side effects.

The high-fiber icing on the cake

When people eat meals higher in fiber, they tend to eat less. Both soluble and insoluble fibers discourage overeating by helping us feel fuller faster (increasing bulk in our stomach and by lowering insulin). One study found people ate smaller lunches after eating high-fiber breakfasts. Fiber may also help cut calories by blocking the digestion of some of the fat, protein, or carbohydrate eaten at the same time. So get your fiber because of all the health benefits.

Flaxseed: the "oat bran" of the new millennium

If you haven't heard of flaxseed yet, trust me you will. I predict flaxseed will be to the 21st century what oat bran was to the 1990s. It is being studied in humans as we speak, mostly for its blood lipid lowering benefits and tumor-reducing properties with some types of cancer.

Dr. Lilian Thompson for the University of Toronto has provided early compelling results that cancer may be reversed—breast cancer size actually decreased—with a daily dose of flaxseed. But Dr. Thompson warns, "We don't have data yet. The study is ongoing." We have to hang tight until more research comes in.

What is it about flaxseed that might be responsible for this? Flaxseed is an extraordinary source of the phytoestrogen called lignins. (Flaxseed contains 75 to 800 times as many lignins as other plant sources.) Lignans also act as antioxidants, protecting healthy cells from chance meetings with free radicals in the body. About 50 percent of the fat in flaxseed is the plant form of omega-3 fatty acids and alpha-linolenic acid. It is possible the fish-based form of omega-3 fatty acids are more powerful in the body, but it appears that the plant form offers benefits as well (such as helping prevent blood clots that might

---

F.Y.I. Flax facts

- **Start by grinding the seeds.** The beneficial components will be more available to your body this way.
- **Keep what you don't use that day in the refrigerator.** Ground flaxseed is highly perishable (lasting only 30 days—and that's if it's refrigerated).
- **Use the seeds instead of the oil.** Although flaxseed oil contains omega-3 fatty acids, it won't contain the beneficial lignans and fiber. (They are both removed in the process of making the oil.)
- **You will find flaxseed (very inexpensive) in bulk bins in health food stores.** If you buy them whole, you will need to store them in the refrigerator and grind them yourself in a spice or coffee grinder one week's supply at a time. Store the unused ground flaxseed in a sealable bag in the refrigerator.
- **It tastes like wheat germ.** Flaxseed has a pleasant nutty taste to it so you can add a little when baking bread, muffins, or when making a smoothie.
- **Try a teaspoon of ground flaxseed a few times a week.** This may be something to consider until more is known on the ideal daily dose.
- **Some people are highly allergic.** Start with a quarter teaspoon and increase the amount gradually if you don't have a reaction.
- **If Flaxseed had a nutrition label, you would see that one teaspoon contains:** 16 calories, 1 g fat, 0.1 g saturated fat, 0.2 g monounsaturated fat, 0.6 g omega-3 fatty acids, 0.9 g fiber (1/3 of which is soluble), 2,200 micrograms total lignans (phytoesterogens).

lead to heart attacks). But even if all of these health benefits fall through, flaxseed is, at the very least, a good source of soluble fiber.

Food Step 5: Keep fat, saturated fat, and animal fat moderate

Researchers are still trying to figure out if and how the amount of fat (as well as the types of fat) in our food changes our risk for breast cancer. It is possible that the fat we eat influences the fatty acid content of breast tissue and this could encourage or discourage certain breast tumors. It has also been reported that a low-fat high-carbohydrate diet seems to decrease breast density, which can make mammograms easier to read. Other researchers believe that if dietary fat influences breast cancer risk, it might actually be more important during our preadult growing years. There does seem to be some evidence that the amount of fat in food affects breast tumorigenesis in mice and rats (*P R Health Sci J*, 1998 Sep;17[3]:273).

I can't really give you specific amounts of fat that are recommended. There is still such uncertainty in this area. However, I can say that a high-fat diet—especially one high in saturated fat—is probably not going to reduce your risk of breast cancer. Whether the ideal level of fat for breast cancer prevention is 30 percent calories from fat or lower is still the question.

Experience has taught me that people who eat diets higher in dietary fat do tend to eat higher amounts of calories. Extra calories over time will certainly encourage extra body fat in some people. And since obesity is believed to increase the risk of breast cancer—especially in postmenopausal women—this would present us yet another reason not to eat a high-fat diet.

What continues to complicate this issue is the various types of fat: saturated, polyunsaturated, and monounsaturated. For example, when two people are eating 30 percent calories from fat, one can be getting it mostly from saturated fat sources while another can be consuming 15 percent of calories from fat from monounsaturated sources, and 8 percent each from saturated and unsaturated fat sources. This might make a big difference in terms of breast cancer risk. A recent French study added to the evidence that saturated fat intake increases breast cancer risk in postmenopausal women (*Eur J Epidemiology*, 1998 Dec;14[8]: 737).

Eat red meat in moderation

Some scientists advise limiting red meat to less than three ounces a day. That barely covers your average quarter pounder (4 ounces raw equals approximately three ounces cooked). That's tough to do in the United States.

A number of studies show that people who eat large portions of red meat develop more cancers (particularly colon and rectal cancers) but also prostate, pancreatic, and breast cancers (Laurence Kolonel, M.D., Ph.D., University of Hawaii).

Red meat contributes saturated fat, which might increase the risk of cancers of the breast as well as the lung, colon and rectum, uterus, and prostate. It is interesting though that poultry (turkey and chicken) hasn't shown an association with cancer in most studies (Laurence Kolonel, M.D., Ph.D., University of Hawaii). Chicken can form HCAs if grilled or fried and fish can also form HCAs. Fish also contains omega-3 fatty acids, which may be helpful in lowering cancer risk.

If you do decide to grill, marinating or microwaving will help

New studies are suggesting that marinating your meat or poultry at least three minutes before cooking may lower HCA formation by 94 to 96 percent. The big bonus is you can't beat the added flavor and tenderizing of the marinades. If you are wondering about the oils often found in marinades, you don't need them for flavor or tendering. In fact, it is best to leave them out—it will help reduce smoking when your meat is grilling. You can get flavor from herbs, spices and vegetables (including the marinade favorites: onion, garlic, ginger, peppers). The tenderizing comes from the added acidic ingredients, such as lemon juice, other juices, wine, beer, or vinegar.

Marinate red meat for up to 24 hours to maximize tenderizing and flavor. The more delicate poultry and seafood, however, is best when marinating for no longer than two hours.

Another thing you can do to reduce possible HCAs from forming on your meat is to precook your meat in the microwave, then grilling or broiling the meat for flavor until done. This can prevent some 90 percent of HCA formation.

Food Step 6: Switch to monounsaturated fats

It looks more and more as if it might be beneficial to switch to mostly monounsaturated fats when you have a choice when cooking at home. Research has been showing that monounsaturated oils, such as olive and canola oil, do not have many cancer-promoting effects (*Journal of the American Dietetic Association*, 97:16, 1997). At the same time, monounsaturated fats are being preferred to saturated fats, more and more, when it comes to blood lipids and heart disease prevention.

Monounsaturated fats do not seem to promote heart disease (plaquing in the arteries) like saturated fats and some polyunsaturated fats appear to. In this book we'll be focusing on the benefit of monounsaturated fats and omega-3 fatty acids in terms of cancer prevention. Just feel good knowing these same steps will help toward heart disease prevention as well.

More on monounsaturated fats

There are two monounsaturated cooking oils to choose from: olive oil and canola oil. I use olive oil for pasta salads, salad dressings, and my Italian and Mediterranean recipes. I use canola oil for oven frying and sautéing. In many baking recipes (some cakes, muffins, brownies, and even pie crust) I switch to canola oil. If the cookie or cake recipe calls for creaming shortening or butter with sugar, then I usually can't switch to canola oil. In that case, I use canola margarine or butter, just less of it.

What's better: olive or canola oil?

At this point, it looks like one isn't necessarily better than the other—they both offer benefits. They both contain monounsaturated fats. But canola oil handles the high heat of oven frying and stir frying better than olive oil. Canola also contributes plant-based omega-3 fatty acids. Olive oil has a pungent flavor while canola has a neutral flavor. This "olive" flavor can either be a good thing or a not so good thing depending on the recipe. It can either complement or compete with the other flavors. Olive oil also contains potentially protective phytochemicals common in olives.

Bigger fish to fry: omega-3 fatty acids

Researchers observed that women from countries with less breast cancer have higher levels of omega-3 fatty acids. Nineteen research papers on carcinogenesis found when omega-3 is added to the diet of test animals, fewer and smaller tumors have been found after cancer-causing chemicals were added to their diet.

You can't discuss omega-3 fatty acids without talking about their alter ego—omega-6 fatty acids (found in corn, safflower, and sunflower oils). Omega-6s compete with omega-3s for control of many biochemical reactions in your body. What happens if you take in a lot more omega-6s than omega-3s? It appears to lead to an overproduction of hormonelike substances (prostaglandins and leukotrienes) which can encourage plaque buildup on artery walls and disrupt the immune system, among other things. Here's the scary part: The typical American diet contains 10 times more omega-6s than omega-3s.

Here are four things you can do to quickly improve your omega-3 to omega-6 ratio:

1. **Eat fish about two times a week.** Omega-3s can be found in all sorts of fish, the fattier the better. My personal favorite fish sources are salmon, canned albacore tuna packed in water, striped bass, and pacific halibut, but you can also find them in anchovies, sardines, herring, bluefish, mackerel, mullet, and shark.

2. **Switch to canola oil, olive oil, or soybean oil for cooking.**

3. **Limit your use of salad dressing, margarine, mayonnaise, and vegetable oils that contain corn, safflower, or sunflower oils.**

4. **Consider adding the following to recipes when possible:** soybeans and soybean products, walnuts, spinach, mustard greens, and flaxseed (all of these are plant sources of omega-3 fatty acids).

Omega-3 fatty acids have been shown to slow or prevent cancerous tumor growth. The two particular cancers that omega-3s may help prevent are colon and breast cancers. One recent laboratory study found that a higher ratio of omega-3 fatty acids to omega-6 fatty acids suppressed human breast cancer growth (Hilda Chamras, UCLA School of Medicine).

A UCLA study is now testing whether omega-3s can help prevent recurrence of cancer in breast cancer survivors. In the meantime, eating fish one to two times a week, working in plant sources of omega-3 fatty acids, and switching to canola or olive oil for cooking are all good ideas for heart disease prevention anyway.

Food Step 7: Drink little or no alcohol

At least 50 studies show that alcohol may play a role in breast cancer risk. Researchers at the Harvard School of Public Health, after pooling the results of six international studies, estimated that drinking two to five alcoholic drinks a day raises a woman's risk of getting breast cancer by more than 40 percent compared to nondrinkers. Women who average one to two drinks a day increase their risk by 16 percent (*Tufts University Health & Nutrition Letter*, April 1998). Put another way, keeping alcohol within recommended limits will prevent up to 20 percent of cases of cancers of the aerodigestive tract, the colon, rectum, and breast (*Food, Nutrition and the Prevention of Cancer: A Global Perspective*, 1997, American Institute for Cancer Research.)

How does alcohol increase risk? Alcohol can increase estrogen levels in the blood. It is even possible that alcohol may encourage tumors to grow faster, as researchers have noticed alcohol has a pronounced effect on women with advanced breast cancer.

Even moderate drinking may be too much. Your risk rises 11 percent if you regularly have one alcoholic drink a day, 24 percent if you drink two drinks, and 40 percent if you drink more than two (Lenore Kohlmeier, professor of epidemiology and nutrition, University of North Carolina in Chapel Hill). The best advice to take if you enjoy alcohol is to limit yourself to three drinks a week.

If you insist on drinking regularly you might strongly consider a trip to the vitamin aisle of your supermarket (or better yet, making sure you eat your fruits and vegetables). Women with the highest daily intake of folic acid (600 mcg/day) were at a 45 percent lower risk of breast cancer, compared with women with the lowest folic acid intake (150 to 299 mcg/day) (Hunter et al., *JAMA* 281[17]:1632-37,1999). You'll find folic acid mostly in leafy green vegetables, legumes, and some fruits (such as oranges).

Food Step 8: Emphasize variety in food choices

One area scientists need to learn more about is the way nutrients interact. Most of the research singles out nutrients or foods as cancer-fighters. But the truth probably is that they each work most effectively in tandem with other nutrients. Eating various foods will give many different nutrients and phytochemicals. Getting these protective nutrients from food instead of pills is probably an important piece of the breast cancer prevention puzzle.

Food Step 9: What are you "weight"ing for?

Excessive food fat and food calories easily becomes body fat. As I discussed previously, body fat may produce extra estrogen, which may help some tumors grow in the breast. A Harvard University study showed that women who gained 44 to 55 pounds after age 18 had almost double the risk of developing breast cancer following menopause, compared with women who had gained only a few pounds.

Are you wearing the fat gene?

Some of us will put on extra pounds much easier than others—even if we have been careful to eat a healthy diet and exercise regularly. I know this from personal experience. I'm almost 40 years old and I'm approximately 40 pounds heavier than I was at 18. I gained 10 impossible-to-lose pounds with each of my two children and another 10 pounds from a hysterectomy. Let me also say that I have eaten very healthy all these years (I was a vegetarian during some of these years). And I have always exercised, except for about six months after my second was born (at that point I had two children under the age of two—need I say more?).

I would have to almost starve myself in order to be thin. My two sisters are exactly the same. We are all just not willing to starve ourselves. We obviously have the genes that favor survival (storing up energy for the next potato famine). In this way, our genes do play a part in how our bodies balance the "calories in" and "energy out" equation. By influencing the amount of body fat and how fat is distributed, genetics can make you more susceptible to gaining weight.

I believe some of us just aren't meant to be thin. I believe there is beauty in curves. I believe "fit" comes in all shapes and sizes. Some of us will add some pounds through the years. What we can do, however, is try to keep these extra pounds as honest as possible—not because we are simply eating too much and exercising too little.

Calories in = calories out

If this equation looks so simple, why is it so hard to maintain? This is the same information we've known and heard about for more than 15 years. However, even with this information we are still trying the latest trendy diets (such as the latest high protein, low carbohydrate craze). The painful truth is this: Americans haven't been increasing the calories "out" side of the equation due to a lifestyle filled with long commutes, computers, television, etc. Add to that the fact that the number of total daily calories has increased by an average of 231 calories per person from 1976 to 1980.

So what can we do about this?

- **Stop dieting.** We know it doesn't work. We know it works against you in the long run. Stop now.
- **Eat when you are hungry and stop when you are comfortable.** When we diet, we force ourselves not to listen to our natural hunger cues. When we do this, we also tend not to listen to our "comfortable" cues and overeat at times. In order to stop overeating and stop obsession about food we need to stop dieting. Some studies show that persons with obesity are unable to determine hunger and satiety for themselves. But dieters who are not eating when hungry, or who are eating too much (bingeing), can disrupt normal satiety cues. If you think you are addicted to dieting or eat compulsively sometimes, do try to get professional help.

- **Exercise!** Steady aerobic exercise (such as walking more than 40 minutes) is one of the best ways to lose body fat. You burn more fat during longer-duration, lower-intensity exercise than you do during shorter exercise periods. Strength training exercises (such as weight training) are also important because they help counteract muscle loss due to aging and help build and maintain muscle. The more lean muscle mass you can preserve, the bigger the "engine" with which to burn calories.

- **Aim for relatively high-carbohydrate, high fiber meals.** Studies indicate that people eating higher carbohydrate diets (including fiber) have a lower percentage of body fat. Studies indicate that women most successful at keeping significant weight loss off over time eat high-carbohydrate, low-fat diets (*Nutrition Updates*, Fall 1999).

- **Change the behaviors that made you overweight in the first place.** Take a look at your eating habits and your daily routine. Do you eat everything on your plate? Do you eat fast? Do you eat most of your food late at night? Do you eat certain foods passed the point of being "comfortable" and why? If you have other issues interfering with your happiness—you'll need to work on these first.

High-fat doesn't help

Ounce for ounce, each gram of dietary fat provides more than twice as many calories as a gram of protein or carbohydrate. Yet when calories are the same, a person eating a high-fat diet tends to store more excess calories as body fat than someone eating a lower-fat diet. Some recent research is even suggesting that carbohydrates and protein are more "satisfying" than fat too.

But eating a very low-fat diet is not the answer either. I think you need some fat in your food to help keep balance with carbohydrates and proteins. Dietary fat also contributes important fat-soluble vitamins (such as vitamin E) and important potentially protective fatty acids (like the omega-3s).

Attitude is everything

It is counterproductive and emotionally dangerous to concentrate on losing pounds to improve appearance or to reach some magical number on the scale. Rather, a healthier approach is to simply focus on health. Let the pounds fall where they may. That's all we can really do.

Is there still a place for dessert?

The first place people "watch it" is with desserts. We think of them as extras. They are merely here for our enjoyment—but that's worth something!

If you love a particular dessert—go ahead and enjoy it occasionally without guilt (and without overeating). This is important. Just knowing you can have something you really want—when you want it—helps some people refrain from overeating their favorite foods when they do finally have them. For all the days in between, keep the tips in "Shopping with a sweet tooth" (Chapter 7, page 130) in mind.

Food Step 10: Get bitten by the fitness bug

I got bitten by the fitness bug many moons ago. It stings at first if you aren't used to it. Getting on the stationary bike after a long day when you would really rather lie on the couch is hard. Writing a check for the dance or exercise class you are taking is sometimes harder. Getting up an hour earlier to take a quick walk before breakfast can be incredibly difficult. Exercise takes up time and sometimes money. But boy, is it worth it!

After a short time (hopefully) you just can't help but start to love lots of things about exercising. Your body feels better, younger, and more energetic. I've noticed that overweight women who start exercising feel better about their bodies (and more attractive) than women who are about the same dress size but who don't exercise. That's worth it alone! That doesn't even begin to mention the long list of health benefits from regular exercise...which brings us to the reason this is one of the "Food Steps to Freedom" in a book about preventing breast cancer.

Some studies have found a reduced risk of breast cancer among women who exercise regularly or who were athletic as adolescents. The evidence appears to be strongest for younger women who exercise. Other studies have found no protective effect at all. One researcher suspects that exercise somehow alters ovarian function, lowering the production of estrogen (the hormone with a suspected link to breast cancer.)

A review of research published in *The Journal of the National Cancer Institute* suggested exercise reduces breast cancer risk both before and after menopause by as much as 60 percent. While a study in the *New England Journal of Medicine* (336: 1269, 1311, 1997) reported that women who exercised at least four hours a week had a 37 percent lower risk of breast cancer than sedentary women. Whether it is a 37-percent or a 60-percent reduced risk, it helps to exercise your body.

It is difficult to measure physical activity of individuals over a lifetime, therefore studying whether exercise decreases the risk of disease is equally as difficult. Some researchers believe if exercise offers protection against breast cancer it is only very modest protection. However, I'll take modest protection over no protection. No matter what, exercise helps us prevent obesity, which may have its own effect on breast cancer risk.

The best advice is this: Try to exercise at least four hours a week—even if it is just walking. A Norwegian study of more than 25,000 women found this reduced breast cancer risk by 37 percent. No matter what the final verdict is with exercise's cancer-preventing powers, it is still a great way to reduce the risk of heart disease, diabetes, stroke, and obesity.

New developments to keep an eye on

Did you get your vitamin D and your dairy today? It is starting to look as if vitamin D (a fat soluble vitamin) may have a link to breast cancer risk reduction. You can worry less about getting enough D if you get a healthy dose of sunshine most of the time. The sunshine is needed by the skin to manufacture vitamin D. How much sun is enough? Usually 10 to 15 minutes a day will get you close to the adequate levels. But how much D is needed to help prevent breast cancer? We don't know yet.

What is the best advice if you are indoors most of the time? Women who get about 200 IU a day (the amount in 2 cups of milk) may lower their risk of breast cancer by about 30 percent. However, because vitamin D is fat soluble, our body can't get rid of excess amounts so it—it is important not to take in too much. In a laboratory study, yogurt (which contains only a very small amount of vitamin D) slowed the growth of breast cancer cells even *after* the active bacterial cultures were removed from the yogurt (*Nutrition and Cancer*, 28, 1, 1997).

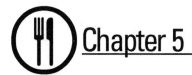 <u>Chapter 5</u>

The Joy of Eating

E ating is one of the greatest pleasures of life. I may be a registered dietitian, but that hasn't stopped me from enjoying food and the grand art of eating, cooking, and feeding others. Food should be enjoyed. If you aren't enjoying the food you are eating, there is something wrong with the food or with you.

Now, I'll admit that along the way I have met people who don't care about the pleasures of eating. To them, food is fuel. They eat simply to survive. It's no surprise that these people are usually very thin (and many smoke). But *most* people—and most women—enjoy eating. This shouldn't change—healthy food should still taste good. If it doesn't, chances are you won't be able to stick to your new healthful dietary habits for long.

If you are choking down a banana in the name of health, for example, please don't. Instead pick fruits you like. If you like berries and it is wintertime, buy them frozen and whip up a quick smoothie. If you love peaches and it is spring, buy them canned in peach juice (they are still pretty good this way).

If you like apples, keep them in the crisper so they taste refreshingly nice and cold. If you like grapes, freeze some and pull them out as an ice-cold snack on a hot afternoon. If you like pears, serve a fresh or canned pear half with a small dollop of cranberry sauce in the scooped out part of the pear as a side dish or dessert.

If the food doesn't taste good, it obviously takes away from the joy of eating. But there is something less obvious that can zap the joy right out of eating—counting. Counting calories, fat grams, or tabulating food group servings—take your pick. If you have to count anything having to do with your meal before, during, or after you eat, it can take the joy not only out of eating, but out of living. Anytime you put yourself in a "counting" mode, day in and day out, you automatically snap into the "dieting" mentality, which often leaves you feeling defeated, deprived, and depressed.

Don't get me wrong, I don't mind *periodic* counting. That's when, every now and then, you check in to see how your average daily food intake compares to certain standards or recommendations. It can be useful as long as it is a checkpoint and not a daily regimen. There are people who, for their continued health, have to count certain nutrients (such as people with diabetes or renal disease). Believe me, one of their greatest challenges (and their dietitian's greatest challenge) is maintaining the joy of eating.

Is it my imagination, or is my body changing its shape?

It's not your imagination if you notice your body is changing as you go through your 30s, 40s, and 50s. For example, after menopause, excess body fat is more likely to be distributed above and around your waist rather than on your hips, buttocks, or thighs. This means your shape may be looking a little more like an apple than the pear shape of your past.

The sad truth is that as we age, body water, bone density, and muscle mass all tend to decrease while body fat increases. We can fight this by keeping our hydration and bone density as high as possible and by maintaining and building our muscle mass as we age.

Maintaining your muscle mass

Muscle mass and muscle strength also tend to decline as you age, because you start losing more and more muscle fibers and nerves that stimulate them. But you enhance your muscle mass through strength training and regular exercise. In terms of diet, you should make sure you are getting enough protein but not too much—In this case, more is not better. The only true way to *build* muscle is to *use* muscle.

Why start strength training?

Anyone can start boosting their muscle mass by doing appropriate strength training exercises two to three times a week. You may have heard of these other terms for strength training: resistance training, weight training, and isotonics. Strength-training exercises usually involve activities that you repeat eight to 12 times in a row while standing or sitting in one place. The exercises pull a muscle (or set of muscles) to exhaustion. This encourages the muscle to grow and improve its tone. Strength training can be done two to three times a week for 30 to 40 minutes each session. Here are four great reasons to start strength training A.S.A.P.:

- Strength training builds muscle mass. Because muscle mass requires *more* calories to sustain itself than body fat, strength training helps raise your metabolic rate.

- Strength training increases bone density so it also helps reduce the risk of osteoporosis.

- The more muscle you have, the less insulin is required to get sugar from the blood to body tissues. Strength training helps reduce your risk of developing diabetes in your later years.
- Strength training can ease the pain of osteoarthritis and may even ease the pain of rheumatoid arthritis.

Stop diets and start getting fit

Most experts and chronic dieters can agree on one thing—dieting doesn't work. When tempted by new diets out there, remember this—quick weight loss tends to break down lean body tissue (muscles and organ tissue). Weight regain tends to put on body fat—exactly the opposite of what we want to happen.

If we could all change our goal from losing weight to gaining health—we would all be better off. To gain health we simply focus on eating healthy and getting regular exercise. To help us do this it is essential we remember two things: you don't have to be thin to be fit and healthy, and a healthy weight is the weight you maintain without too much trouble.

Minimizing weight gain by being in a "health" mindset

If you focus on losing pounds you immediately put yourself in a dieting mindset where you are more likely to fall into the weighing-yourself-daily failure trap. Change your focus to being and feeling healthy. I believe in eating right and exercising for the health of it...and let the pounds fall where they may. The one area you might need to look at more closely though is changing the habits that might be leading you to excess weight.

Do you have any unhealthy eating habits? Take the quiz below and find out:

1. Do you snack on sweets and chips more than fresh fruit and vegetables?
2. Do you eat everything on your plate every time, thinking you would be wasting food if you didn't?
3. Do you find yourself eating when you aren't really hungry because you are under stress, bored, angry, or upset? (Research indicates that using food to soothe feelings may be one big reason many people who lose weight gain it back.)
4. Do you think you are being "bad" when you have your favorite foods? Do you think you must give them up in order to lose weight?
5. Do you sometimes sit down for a small snack and end up eating a whole box of cookies, bag of chips, or small carton of ice cream?
6. Do you sometimes let yourself get too hungry because you are trying to lose weight by not eating, even when you are hungry?
7. Do you eat a lot of food late at night?

Now, trade the destructive habits above in for the healthful habits below:

1. Do you eat when you are hungry and stop when you are comfortable (not full)?
2. Do you eat mostly plant foods, making sure you eat at least five servings of fruits and vegetables every day?
3. Do you drink alcohol only on occasion (or not at all)? When you do drink, do you keep it to no more than one drink a day?
4. If there is a certain food you *really* want, and you are physically hungry, do you have it in a small but satisfying portion?
5. Are you trying to eat more fiber-rich foods (fruits, vegetables, whole grains) and more balanced meals and snacks, including some protein and fat (mostly monounsaturated fat) because this generally makes meals more satisfying and staves off hunger longer?

6. Do you eat light at night, knowing you will be more comfortable sleeping if you aren't full, waking up hungry and ready to start your day?

7. Do you exercise regularly because you know it is important for your overall health?

8. Do you avoid distractions—such as reading or watching television—when you eat? Do you try to eat slowly and savor the taste of your food?

9. Do you find other ways to comfort yourself when you are bored, stressed, angry or upset? (Such as going for a walk, calling a friend, listening to some uplifting music, or taking a bubble bath?) Don't ignore your feelings—Find healthier ways of dealing with them. It's easier said than done, but get professional counselling with this if you need it.

10. Do you weigh yourself only when in doctors' offices because you know that the numbers on a scale really don't matter? What matters most is your overall health and how you feel.

Foods to maximize

If it seems like you are constantly being told what *not* to eat: "Cut back on fat and calories," "limit sugar and sodium," "eat less saturated fat and cholesterol," and on and on... But there is a better way of looking at this same nutritional picture.

Instead of dwelling on what to cut out, focus on what is *missing*. The more we learn about health and nutrition, the more researchers realize that fruits and vegetables are a vital key to health and vitality. This attitude change will do more for you (and your children) in terms of your physical, nutritional, and emotional health than following a set of rules about what not to eat. All it takes is a quick look at "10 Food Steps to Freedom" and you will be reminded of all the foods we need to eat more of.

To refresh your memory, here are a list of things to maximize in your diet:

- **Maximize the omega-9 fatty acids which are also the monounsaturated fats** (such as olive oil and canola oil).
- **Maximize omega-3 fatty acids such as fish, and other plant foods that contain alpha-linolenic acid.** The body can partially convert alpha-linolenic acid to one of the omega-3 fatty acids.
- **Maximize whole grains and whole grain products, soybean products, and beans** for fiber and important phytochemicals.
- **Maximize the most nutrient-packed fruits, vegetables, and juices** for important antioxidants, vitamins, minerals, phytochemicals and fiber.

Maximize your calorie burning

Should you eat fewer calories? You could, but that isn't very much fun. Your body needs more of various nutrients as you age anyway. If you eat less, you aren't likely to be getting more of these nutrients (such as calcium, vitamin D, antioxidants, vitamin B-12, zinc, etc.) And there are so many other health benefits to the suggestions below. You are truly better off burning more calories rather than eating a lot less. Here's how to burn more calories:

1. **Exercising.** Exercising, in general, helps increase the number of calories you burn in a day. Of course we know we burn the extra calories *while* we exercise, but some new evidence suggests we even burn extra calories *after* we exercise (possibly four to 12 hours after exercise.)

   When you just begin to exercise regularly, you use mostly glucose (carbohydrate) as your main fuel during aerobic exercise. Once you get into a regular exercise program and your body becomes more fit, your body will start to burn *more* fat for the extra energy you need while you are exercising. Generally after exercising 20 minutes, the experienced exerciser is probably primarily burning fat for fuel. Go for at least 20 minutes of valuable fat-burning time, then, you want to strive for those aerobic workouts that go for at least 40 minutes.

2. **Build muscle to burn more calories.** Muscle cells burn more calories at rest than fat cells do. How many calories are we talking about? About 70 percent of the calories you burn in a day are due to the metabolic activity of your lean body mass (muscle). If you want to build muscle tissue instead of fat tissue, exercise has to be part of your plan. For best results use a combination of aerobic conditioning and strength training, especially during and after menopause.

3. **Eat breakfast.** Your metabolism (the rate at which the body burns calories) may slow down if you go long periods without eating. It shuts down to conserve fuel. One of the biggest gaps in eating is night time, when we sleep. If you are one of those people who isn't hungry right when you wake up, drink a small glass of juice or milk then pack some food to bring with you wherever you go. An hour of two later when your hunger kicks in, you will be prepared.

4. **Eat small, frequent meals through the day...and eat light at night.** Each time you eat, you set your body's digestive process in motion. Each time you start it up, you burn calories. The more frequently you eat, the more calories you burn just by digesting your food.

5. **Burn more calories digesting high-carbohydrate foods.** Your body uses more energy (burns more calories) to metabolize carbohydrates than it does to break down dietary fat. For example, if you eat 100 high-fat potato chip calories in excess of your calorie needs, about 97 of the 100 calories will probably end up as fat storage. But if you eat 100 higher carbohydrate calories as a baked potato, 77 calories will probably deposited as fat (your body burned 23 calories to digest, convert, and store those mostly carbohydrate calories).

I'm eating healthful and exercising, so why am I not losing weight?

If you are exercising regularly and strength training as well, you are probably adding muscle weight while decreasing some body fat. Remember, muscle weighs more than body fat. Your weight could very well stay the same even though you are building muscle and losing body fat. Keep in mind—you *are* healthier for it.

You could also take a look at portion sizes. It is possible, even if you are choosing healthful foods, that the portions may be too large for your caloric needs. If you keep this up, you won't see any actual lost "pounds." Or, if you eat out often, you may be eating more calories or fat grams than you realize.

Making the switch

Most of us are quite aware that we should be eating less fat, eating more fruits and vegetables, and exercising more. The truth is that it just isn't that simple. *Knowing* we should be doing it and actually *doing it* are two very different things indeed.

Let's talk about what it might take to just do it. There are four main stages in accepting loss—denial, anger, grief, acceptance. In the same way, change doesn't come easy. However, there are stages of change too, according to James Prochaska, Ph.D., a psychologist and head of Health Promotion Partnership at the University of Rhode Island and author of *Changing for Good* (William Morrow and Company, 1994).

Gradually, people become more focused to the disadvantages of the old behavior and the advantages of change. All of this takes time. People talk about willpower being the essential ingredient for change. But willpower or commitment by itself, isn't enough. Dr. Prochaska, and many others, believe you need to *prepare* for change.

Stages of change

1. **Precontemplation.** You have no current intention of changing. You might even feel a situation is hopeless. You use denial and defensiveness to keep from going forward. Consciousness-raising may help move you forward at this stage.

2. **Contemplation.** You accept or realize you have a problem and you start to seriously think about changing it. A lot of people get stuck at this stage. They might be waiting for absolute certainty (which rarely exists), a magical moment of change (you make your own magic), or they might be secretly hoping for another way out without having to change their behavior. More consciousness-raising and learning more about the subject can help at this stage.

3. **Preparation.** You are starting to pull yourself in a new direction. You plan to take action within a month. You are starting to think more about the future than the past, and more about the positives of the new behavior than about the negatives of the old one. Telling others about your intentions and developing a plan for action can help at this stage.

4. **Action.** You start the new behavior. Rewarding yourself and making your environment as change-friendly as possible helps at this stage.

5. **Maintenance.** You are sticking with your new behavior. Remind yourself that maintenance is an ongoing process that is often more difficult to achieve than the action stage. Maintenance is often blindsighted by three things: overconfidence, daily temptation, and blaming yourself for lapses. Expect those three common challenges to maintenance. In terms of relapses, just accept ahead of time that there will be some. Plan to learn from each relapse. Have a plan to help avoid or minimize the daily temptations you may have in your life. Keep going with your strategies for the action stage

(commitment, reward, a change-friendly environment, surrounding yourself with people who help and support your change, and so forth).

The "M" word: motivation

According to Dr. Prochaska, there are two ways to get more motivated: Make a single motive extremely important and/or increase the number of motives. That's what trying to prevent breast cancer does for many of us: It increases the number of motives. Surrounding ourselves with people who believe in and applaud our changes adds some motivation.

If at first you don't succeed...

On average, the same New Year's resolutions are made three years in a row. Sometimes people jump to one of the later stages when they really haven't prepared themselves for change. Many end up going back to their old habits, thinking they have failed because they are too weak. The truth is most people lapse at some point. Lapsing, in a way, is a part of the process of change. Where people usually go wrong is not taking action again. Action followed by relapse is better than no action at all. Use your experience to help yourself the next time you get back on the horse. Remind yourself that you have more than one chance to change.

In order to help you prepare, take action, and maintain these healthful diet changes, you will find practical tips and information in the next three chapters. See Chapter 6 for recipes, Chapter 7 for practical supermarket advice, and Chapter 8 for the do's and don'ts of dining out.

 ## Chapter 6

The Recipes You
Cannot Live Without

This chapter contains the recipes that will help you follow the "10 Food Steps to Freedom." Most of the recipes will help you follow the first four—eating more of the powerful fruits and vegetables and eating more fiber.

We know we should be eating more fruits, vegetables and beans, but we can't seem to make it happen. I wanted to put together quick recipes that were packed with fruits, vegetables and beans, but tasty enough that you actually craved eating them. I know, it sounds strange to actually crave fruits and vegetables. But I believe deep down your body knows what it needs. It will want you to make many of these recipes again and again.

This chapter is not meant to be the answer to all your recipe woes. It is just a sampling to get you started. I have written several other cookbooks that will also come in handy: *The Recipe Doctor* (a collection of columns from my national column, "The Recipe Doctor"), and *Chez Moi* (lightening up recipes from famous restaurants).

(**Please note:** The following is a key to the abbreviations used in the recipes: tablespoon [tbs.], teaspoon [tsp.], gram [g], milligram [mg], ounces [oz.], pound [lb.], and retinol [vitamin A] equivalents [RE].)

Super salad recipes

 ## Super Side Salad

Makes 1 serving.

- 2 cups lettuce of your choice, shredded or chopped (fresh spinach leaves will add even more nutrients and phytochemicals)
- 3 cherry tomatoes
- 1/4 cup canned kidney beans, drained and rinsed
- 1/4 cup grated carrot
- 1/4 cup raw chopped broccoli florets
- 3 tbs. reduced-fat Italian dressing a or similar dressing (I like Wishbone's Olive Oil Vinaigrette or Seven Seas "1/3 Less-Fat Red Wine Vinegar & Oil.")

1. Arrange lettuce in individual salad bowl or plate.
2. Arrange tomatoes, beans, carrot, broccoli over the top.
3. Drizzle with your favorite low calorie dressing.

Per serving: 151 calories, 5.5 g protein, 21 g carbohydrate, 7.5 g fat, 0.5 g saturated fat, 3 mg cholesterol, 7.5 g fiber, 400-600 mg sodium. Calories from fat: 29 percent.

1,176 RE vitamin A (147 percent RDA).
74 mg vitamin C (123 percent RDA).
2.5 mg vitamin E (31 percent RDA).

Super Chinese Chicken Salad

Makes 4 large servings.

- 4 chicken breasts, skinless and boneless
- 3 cups low-sodium chicken broth
- 2 1/2 cups raw broccoli florets, (cut large florets into bite sized pieces)
- 1 1/2 cups green beans or Chinese snow peas, remove stems and cut into bite size pieces
- 2 carrots, grated
- 4 green onions, thinly sliced diagonally
- 3 cups finely shredded iceberg lettuce (or other lettuce)
- 1 package uncooked ramen noodle soup (discard the flavoring packet)

Dressing:

- 3 tbs. honey
- 1/4 cup orange juice
- 3 tbs. seasoned rice vinegar
- 1 tbs. sesame oil
- 1/2 tbs. sugar
- 1-2 tbs. toasted sesame seeds or almond slices or slivers (Toast by heating over medium-low heat in small, nonstick sauce or pan, stirring frequently, until lightly brown.)

1. Poach chicken breasts in chicken broth in medium sized saucepan over medium-low heat until cooked through-out (about 15 minutes). Remove from broth and let cool.
2. While chicken is cooking, place broccoli and green beans in microwave-safe covered dish with 1/4 cup water and microwave on high for about 4 minutes or until just barely cooked but still crisp. Drain vegetables and let cool.
3. Cut chicken diagonally into thin strips. In serving bowl, toss chicken with broccoli, green beans, carrot, green onions, iceberg lettuce, and ramen noodles (break into small pieces as you add in).

4. In small food processor or blender (or use a covered jar or a wire whisk with a small deep bowl) blend dressing ingredients until smooth. Pour over salad ingredients and toss to coat well. Sprinkle almonds or sesame seeds over the top.

Per serving: (using *regular* ramen soup noodles) 390 calories, 32 g protein, 41 g carbohydrate, 11 g fat, 2 g saturated fat, 68 mg cholesterol, 5.5 g fiber, 200 mg sodium. Calories from fat: 25 percent.

1152 RE vitamin A (144 percent RDA).
73 mg vitamin C (122 percent RDA).
1.1 mg vitamin E (14 percent RDA).

 # Super Pasta Salad

Makes 6 to 8 servings.
- 4 cups dried rotelle pasta (or other shaped pasta)
- 4 cups raw broccoli florets
- 6-8 green onions, finely chopped
- 4 Roma tomatoes (or 4 vine ripened tomatoes), coarsely chopped
- 1 pasilla chili pepper, finely chopped (a green pepper may be substituted)
- 15-20 pimento stuffed Spanish olives
- 1 cup fresh basil leaves, torn into bite-sized pieces
- 1 cup firmly packed grated reduced-fat sharp cheddar cheese (4 oz.)

Dressing:
- 1 packet Good Seasons Caesar salad dressing
- 2 tbs. seasoned rice vinegar
- 3 tbs. apple juice
- 1 tbs. olive oil

1. Cook pasta in boiling water according to package directions until tender.
2. Microwave broccoli florets in 1/4 cup water on high just until lightly cooked (about 3-4 minutes).
3. In large serving bowl, toss drained broccoli and cooled noodles with green onions, tomatoes, chili pepper, whole olives, basil leaf pieces, and grated cheese.
4. To make dressing, add packet powder to covered jar along with vinegar, apple juice, and olive oil. Cover and shake vigorously to blend. Pour over salad ingredients and toss to blend.

Per serving (if serving 6): 385 calories, 17 g protein, 62 g carbohydrate, 8 g fat, 2 g saturated fat, 13 mg cholesterol, 5.5 g fiber, 452 mg sodium. Calories from fat: 19 percent.

224 RE vitamin A (28 percent RDA).
105 mg vitamin C (175 percent RDA).
1.75 mg vitamin E (22 percent RDA).

 # Ramen Cabbage Salad

Makes 6 servings.
- 1/3 cup slivered or sliced almonds
- 2 tbs. sesame seeds
- 6 cups shredded cabbage
- 4 green onions, finely chopped (white portion and half of green)
- 1 cup canned black beans, drained and rinsed
- 1 package Ramen Noodle Soup

Dressing:
- 3 tbs. honey
- Ramen seasoning packet
- 2 tbs. apple juice
- 3 tbs. rice vinegar
- 1 tbs. sesame oil

1. Toast sesame seeds and almonds separately by laying them in a single layer of a pan and broiling carefully until lightly brown. Set both aside. Put cabbage, almonds, sesame seeds, onions, and beans in serving bowl. Add Ramen noodles after crumbling them into small pieces with your hands.
2. Mix dressing ingredients well with wire whisk in small bowl. Drizzle over the cabbage mixture and toss. (Make sure you mix dressing just before tossing with salad ingredients.

Per serving: 230 calories, 7 g protein, 31 g carbohydrate, 10 g fat, 2 g saturated fat, 0 mg cholesterol, 5 g fiber, 660 mg sodium. Calories from fat: 39 percent.

11 RE vitamin A (1.5 percent RDA).
24 mg vitamin C (40 percent RDA).
3.15 mg vitamin E (40 percent RDA).

 ## Carrots with Apricots

Makes 4 servings.
- 1 cup dried apricots
- 3 cups carrots, cut into 1/2-inch rounds
- 1/4 cup orange juice or water
- 1 tsp. butter or canola margarine
- A pinch of sugar
- Chopped fresh parsley or parsley flakes for garnish

1. Add apricots to microwave-safe small bowl and cover with hot water. Soak 1 1/2 hours to soften or microwave on high for 2 minutes. Drain, pat apricots dry, and cut into julienne strips.
2. In a skillet or frying pan with a tightly fitting lid, combine carrots, orange juice or water, butter and sugar. Cover and cook over medium heat for 12 to 15 minutes

or until carrots are tender. Stir occasionally to prevent sticking. Stir in apricots and heat through. Serve garnished with parsley.

Per serving: 147 calories, 2.5 g protein, 34.5 g carbohydrate, 1.3 g fat, 0.6 g saturated fat, 2.5 mg cholesterol, 5.5 g fiber, 90 mg sodium. Calories from fat: 8 percent.

3,118 RE vitamin A (390 percent RDA).
11 mg vitamin C (18 percent RDA).
1.2 mg vitamin E (15 percent RDA).

 # Easy 3-Bean Salad

Makes 8 servings.

- 15-oz. can kidney beans (less salt variety if available), rinsed and drained
- 15-oz. can garbanzo beans (less salt variety if available), rinsed and drained
- 15 oz. can white beans (such as Cannellini), rinsed and drained
- 2 carrots, grated
- 1/2 cup chopped onion
- 2 cups broccoli, slightly steamed or microwaved
- 3/4 cup bottled vinaigrette salad dressing of choice (choose one using olive oil or canola oil and around 5 g of fat per 2 tbs. serving)

1. Toss the first six ingredients together in a serving bowl.
2. Add dressing to bean mixture and toss well.
3. Refrigerate until needed.

Per serving: 233 calories, 10.5 g protein, 38 g carbohydrate, 4.7 g fat, .5 g saturated fat, 0 mg cholesterol, 9.3 g fiber, 385 mg sodium. Calories from fat: 18 percent.

542 RE vitamin A (68 percent RDA).
25 mg vitamin C (42 percent RDA).
1.2 mg vitamin E (15 percent RDA).

 # Broccoli Salad

Makes 10 servings.

- 7 cups chopped fresh broccoli, loosely packed (about 1 1/2 16-oz. bags if using frozen cut broccoli)
- 8 slices Louis Rich turkey bacon, cooked crisp and crumbled
- 1 cup cashews, peanuts or pecan pieces
- 1/2 cup raisins
- 1/2 medium red onion, finely chopped
- 1/4 cup canola mayonnaise (Best Foods [Hellman's] or Miracle Whip can also be used)
- 1/3 cup fat free or light sour cream
- 2 tbs. sugar
- 2 tbs. sherry vinegar (other vinegar may be used)
- Seasoning salt (optional)

1. Add broccoli to large, covered, microwave-safe dish with 1/2 cup water. Microwave until broccoli is crisp-tender (about 5-7 minutes). Drain the broccoli and let cool.
2. In a large bowl, combine the cooled broccoli, crumbled bacon, nuts, raisins and red onion.
3. In a small bowl, stir together the mayonnaise, sour cream, sugar and vinegar until smooth. Add seasoning salt to taste if desired.
4. Pour the dressing over the broccoli mixture; toss to coat the broccoli mixture with dressing. Cover and chill the salad 2 to 24 hours. Stir the salad before serving.

Per serving (if 10 per recipe): 209 calories, 6.5 g protein, 19.5 g carbohydrate, 13 g fat, 2 g saturated fat, 10 mg cholesterol, 3 g fiber, 234 mg sodium. Calories from fat: 50 percent.

111 RE vitamin A (14 percent RDA).
58 mg vitamin C (97 percent RDA).
1.7 mg vitamin E (21 percent RDA).

Super soup recipes

 ## Homestyle Lentil Soup

Makes 8 servings.
- 3 medium onions, diced
- 4 fresh garlic cloves, minced
- 3 tbs. olive oil
- 8 cups chicken broth
- 1 lb. dried lentils, washed and picked over
- 2 potatoes, washed and diced
- 4 Roma tomatoes, quartered
- 2 large carrots, diced
- 2 tbs. fresh oregano leaves, finely chopped (or 1 1/2 tsp. dried oregano leaves)
- 3/4 tsp. freshly ground black pepper
- Salt to taste

1. In a large pot, sauté the onion and garlic in olive oil until lightly browned. Add all other ingredients and bring to a boil.
2. Cover and let soup boil for 15 minutes. Reduce heat to a simmer and let cook 1/2 to 1 hour.

Per serving: 368 calories, 23.5 g protein, 55 g carbohydrate, 7.3 g fat, 1 g saturated fat, 0 g cholesterol, 10.5 g fiber, 790 mg sodium. Calories from fat: 17 percent.

547 RE vitamin A (68 percent RDA).
26.5 mg vitamin C (44 percent RDA).
1.6 mg vitamin E (20 percent RDA).

Chicken Tortilla Soup

Makes 5 servings.

- 3/4 tsp. olive oil
- 2 boneless chicken breasts, cut into bite-sized chunks
- 1/2 cup chopped green onions
- 2 garlic cloves, minced or crushed
- 1/2 tsp. chili powder
- 2 tbs. lime juice (lemon juice can be substituted)
- 2 14-oz. cans chicken broth (use reduced-sodium broth if available)
- 1 cup chunky salsa
- 1 1/2 cups frozen corn
- 1 15-oz. can 50 percent less salt kidney beans, drained
- 5 oz. Guiltless Gourmet Chili & Lime Baked Tortilla Chips (or regular tortilla chips)
- 1/2 cup grated reduced-fat jack cheese

1. Heat oil over medium heat in large nonstick saucepan. Add chicken and cook, stirring frequently until chicken is slightly browned.
2. Add onions, garlic, chili powder, and lime juice. Cook for 2 minutes. Add broth, salsa, corn, and beans. Stir, cover pan, and bring to boil. Reduce to simmer and cook for 10 minutes.
3. Crumble tortilla chips and put 1 oz. worth into the bottom of each large soup bowl. Ladle soup into each bowl and sprinkle cheese over the top.

Per serving: 363 calories, 24.5 g protein, 56 g carbohydrate, 4.5 g fat, 2 g saturated fat, 34 mg cholesterol, 11 g fiber, 1490 mg sodium (will be much less if reduced-sodium broth is used). Calories from fat: 11 percent.

120 RE vitamin A (15 percent RDA).
25 mg vitamin C (40 percent RDA).
0.5 mg vitamin E (6 percent RDA).

Carotene Crock Pot Stew

Makes about 6 servings.

- 1 pound lean beef stew meat, cut in 1-inch cubes (chicken, turkey, lean pork, or even tofu may be substituted)
- 1/4 cup flour
- 1/2 tsp. salt
- 1/4 tsp. white or black pepper
- 3/4 cup low sodium beef broth
- 1/2 tsp. Worcestershire sauce
- 4 cloves garlic, minced or pressed
- 1/2 tsp. paprika
- 1 tsp. *fines herbes* blend (optional)
- 3 cups sliced carrots (about 3 small)
- 3 cups diced or bite size sweet potatoes (about 2 small)
- 1 onion, coarsely chopped
- 14 1/2-oz. can Ready-Cut Mexican/Italian seasoned stewed tomatoes

1. Place meat in crock pot. Mix flour, salt and pepper and pour over meat; stir to coat meat well with flour.
2. Add all remaining ingredients and stir to mix well. Cover and cook on low about 10 hours (on high for about 4 hours).
3. Stir stew thoroughly before serving.

Per serving: 209 calories, 20 g protein, 24.5 g carbohydrate, 3.7 g fat, 1 g saturated fat, 39 mg cholesterol, 4 g fiber, 418 mg sodium. Calories from fat: 5 percent.

1,880 RE vitamin A (235 percent RDA).
24 mg vitamin C (40 percent RDA).
0.8 mg vitamin E (10 percent RDA).

Cream of Cruciferous Soup

Makes 3 large soup servings.

- 1 envelope Lipton Onion Recipe Secrets Soup Mix
- 3 cups water
- 2 cups coarsely chopped raw cauliflower
- 2 cups coarsely chopped raw broccoli
- 4 garlic cloves, minced or pressed
- 2 cups raw Brussels sprout halves
- 1/4 cup Wondra quick-mixing flour
- 1 1/2 cups low fat milk
- 3 tbs. grated parmesan cheese or grated reduced-fat sharp cheddar cheese (optional)

1. Add onion soup mix envelope to medium sized saucepan. Stir in 3 cups water, cauliflower, broccoli, and garlic. Bring to boil over medium heat, stirring occasionally. Cover saucepan and reduce heat to low. Simmer, stirring occasionally, for about 10 minutes or until broccoli and cauliflower are tender. Remove from heat and let cool 5 minutes.
2. While cauliflower and broccoli are cooking, microwave Brussels sprout halves in 1/2 cup of water on high in a microwave-safe covered dish until tender (about 8 minutes).
3. Add slightly cooled onion soup and vegetable mixture and Wondra flour to blender and mix until blended. Pour mixture back into saucepan and stir in milk and Brussels sprouts. Cook over medium-low heat, uncovered, for 5 minutes or until slightly thickened.
4. Ladle into large soup bowls and sprinkle a tbs. of cheese over the top of each serving if desired. (**Note:** To reduce the sodium, use half of one onion soup envelope instead of a full envelope.)

Per serving: 190 calories, 10 g protein, 32 g carbohydrate, 3 g fat, 2 g saturated fat, 9 mg cholesterol, 6.5 g fiber, 925 mg sodium. Calories from fat: 13 percent.

213 RE vitamin A (27 percent RDA).

138 mg vitamin C (230 percent RDA).

0.9 mg vitamin E (11 percent RDA).

 5-Bean Savory Soup

Makes 8 servings.

- 1 tbs. butter or canola margarine
- 2 onions, chopped
- 1/2 tsp. ground sage
- 1/2 tsp. thyme
- 1/4 tsp. black pepper
- 49-oz. can 1/3 less-sodium chicken broth
- 14.5-oz. can stewed tomatoes
- 10.5-oz. can beef consommé
- 15-oz. can 50-percent less-salt kidney beans, drained and rinsed (1 3/4cup)
- 8.5-oz. can lima beans, drained and rinsed
- 15-oz. can 50 percent less-salt black beans, drained and rinsed (1 3/4 cup)
- 15-oz. can great Northern beans, drained and rinsed (1 3/4 cup)
- 1/2 cup fresh green beans, stemmed and cut into bite size pieces
- 3 tbs. fresh chopped chives (or 1 tbs. dried chives)
- 1/2 cup grated parmesan cheese

1. Heat a large nonstick saucepan or soup kettle over medium heat. Add butter and onion and sauté, stirring frequently, until onion is nicely browned.
2. Add in sage, thyme, and black pepper and stir.
3. Stir in chicken broth, tomatoes, beef consommé, assorted beans, green beans, and chives.
4. Bring to gentle boil. Reduce heat to simmer, cover, and let cook 45 minutes to 1 hour to blend flavors. Ladle

into serving bowls and sprinkle parmesan cheese over the top.

Per serving: 274 calories, 18.5 g protein, 39 g carbohydrate, 4.8 g fat, 3 g saturated fat, 9 mg cholesterol, 15 g fiber, 950 mg sodium. Calories from fat: 16 percent.

75 RE Vitamin A (9 percent RDA).
15 mg Vitamin C (25 percent RDA).
0.6 mg Vitamin E (7 percent RDA).

 # Super Minestrone Soup

Makes 5 large dinner servings.

- 5 cups low-sodium beef broth (from packet reconstituted with water or canned)
- 3 carrots, diced
- 3 large outer celery stalks, sliced at a diagonal
- 1 onion, chopped
- 3 to 4 cloves garlic, minced or pressed
- 1 tsp. dried basil, crushed
- 1/2 tsp. dried oregano, crushed
- 1/4 tsp. pepper
- 15-oz. can red kidney beans, drained and rinsed (or great northern beans)
- 15-oz. can Italian style stewed tomatoes (or regular stewed tomatoes)
- 2 cups zucchini pieces (zucchini halved lengthwise and sliced
- 1/2 cup tiny shell macaroni (or similar shaped pasta)
- 4 tbs. freshly grated parmesan cheese (optional)

1. In a large saucepan combine broth, carrot, celery, onion, garlic, basil, oregano, and pepper. Bring to a boil; reduce heat. Cover; simmer for 15 minutes.
2. Stir in beans, tomatoes, zucchini, and macaroni. Return to boiling, cover, and reduce heat to simmer.

Cook 10 minutes more or until vegetables are tender.

3. Serve into serving bowls and sprinkle parmesan cheese over the top of each if desired.

Per serving: 228 calories, 13.5 g protein, 38.5 g carbohydrate, 2.5 g fat, 1.3 g saturated fat, 0 mg cholesterol, 10.5 fiber, 618 mg sodium. Calories from fat: 9 percent.

1,287 RE vitamin A (161 percent RDA).
27 mg vitamin C (44 percent RDA).
1 mg vitamin E (12 percent RDA).

 # Quick Vegetable Ramen Soup

Makes 2 servings.

- 1 package (3 oz.) ramen noodle soup (low-fat if possible)
- 3 cups water
- 2 carrots, thinly sliced
- 2 celery stalks, thinly sliced
- 1 cup sliced fresh mushrooms
- 1 or 2 green onions, white and part green, chopped

Boil water in medium sized saucepan. Add noodles, seasoning packet, and vegetables. Simmer at least 5 minutes or until vegetables are tender. **Note:** You can cut the sodium in half by only adding half of the seasoning packet.

Per serving: 230 calories, 6 g protein, 37 g carbohydrate, 7 g fat, 3.5 g saturated fat, 0 mg cholesterol, 3.5 g fiber, 863 mg sodium. Calories from fat: 27 percent.

2,035 RE vitamin A (254 percent RDA).
13 mg vitamin C (22 percent RDA).
0.7 mg vitamin E (9 percent RDA).

Chicken Matzo Ball Soup

Makes about 6 hearty soup servings.

Matzo balls:

- 1 tbs. canola oil
- 2 tbs. chicken broth (from soup mixture)
- 1 egg
- 6 tbs. fat-free egg substitute
- 3/4 cup matzo meal
- 1 tsp. salt or less (optional)
- Nonstick cooking spray

Other ingredients:

- 6 green onions, white and part green, chopped
- 6 celery stalks, sliced
- 5 carrots, sliced
- 1 49-oz. can chicken broth (1/3 less-sodium types are available)
- 2 cups water
- 1 tsp. parsley flakes
- 1/2 tsp. sage
- 1/2 tsp. summer savory
- 2 chicken thighs, skinless
- 2 chicken breasts, skinless

1. Start by making the matzo balls. Blend canola oil, 2 tbs. broth, egg, and egg substitute together. Add matzo meal and salt (if desired) and blend well. Mix until uniform (add a tbs. of broth if needed). Cover mixing bowl and place in refrigerator for 15 minutes.
2. Spray bottom of large soup pot with no-stick cooking spray. Add onions, celery, carrots, broth, water, spices, and chicken. Bring to a boil. Reduce flame to a high simmer.
3. Form matzo ball mixture into about 12, 1-inch balls. Drop them into the gently boiling water. Cover pot

and cook 30-40 minutes. Remove chicken pieces and let cool. Once cool to the touch, tear off chicken into bite-sized pieces. Add chicken pieces back to soup pot.

Per serving: 253 calories, 23.5 g protein, 23 g carbohydrate, 7.5 g fat, 1.2 g saturated fat, 76 mg cholesterol, 3 g fiber, 870 mg sodium. Calories from fat: 27 percent.

1,717 RE vitamin A (215 percent RDA).
10 mg vitamin C (17 percent RDA).
1.5 mg vitamin E (19 percent RDA).

Power pasta recipes

 ## Power Pesto Pasta

Makes 4 servings.

- 1 cup firmly packed fresh spinach leaves (with stems removed)
- 1 cup firmly packed fresh basil leaves
- 1/2 cup grated parmesan cheese
- 1/4 cup toasted pinenuts or walnuts (Toast nuts by heat in nonstick frying pan or saucepan over medium-low heat, stirring frequently, until lightly browned.)
- 1/4 tsp. salt
- 2 cloves garlic, minced or pressed
- 1 tbs. olive oil
- 3 tbs. low-fat or reduced-fat mayonnaise (1/2 tbs. canola mayo plus 1 1/2 tbs. fat-free sour cream can also be used)
- 4 cups cooked and drained noodles
- 2 cups lightly cooked broccoli florets (steam or microwave until tender)
- 2 cups lightly cooked carrot coins (steam or microwave until tender)

1. Combine spinach and basil leaves, parmesan, pinenuts, salt, garlic, olive oil and mayonnaise in food processor and pulse until pesto texture is formed (a lumpy paste). Add a 1 tbs. or two of milk if needed.
2. Toss with noodles and vegetables. Reheat mixture in large saucepan over low heat if needed.

Per serving: 403 calories, 16.5 g protein, 55 g carbohydrate, 14 g fat, 3.5 g saturated fat, 12 mg cholesterol, 6 g fiber, 500 mg sodium. Calories from fat: 31 percent.

2,139 RE vitamin A (267 percent RDA).
50 mg vitamin C (82 percent RDA).
2 mg vitamin E (25 percent RDA).

Super Kraft Macaroni and Cheese

Makes 4 servings.

- 1 box Kraft White Cheddar Macaroni and Cheese
- 1 1/2 tbs. butter or canola margarine
- 3 tbs. light sour cream
- 1/4 cup low fat milk
- 1/2 cup grated reduced fat sharp cheddar cheese
- 2 cups broccoli florets, steamed or cooked in microwave until tender
- 2 cups carrot coins (slices), steamed or cooked in microwave until tender

1. Boil 6 cups of water. Stir in macaroni from mix. Boil rapidly, stirring occasionally until tender (7 to 10 minutes). Drain well and return to pan. (While macaroni is cooking, you can steam or microwave the vegetables if you haven't already.)
2. Add butter, sour cream, milk, and cheese sauce mix to pan with macaroni noodles. Mix well and stir in grated cheddar cheese and cooked vegetables.

Per serving: 339 calories, 13.5 g protein, 47.5 g carbohydrate, 10.5 g fat, 5.5 g saturated fat, 32 mg cholesterol, 4 g fiber, 606 mg sodium. Calories from fat: 28 percent.

2,100 RE vitamin A (265 percent RDA).
63 mg vitamin C (106 percent RDA).
0.7 mg vitamin E (9 percent RDA).

 Red, White, and Green Lasagna

Makes 8 servings.
- 9 wide strips of lasagna pasta (about 8 oz. uncooked)
- 1 1/2 cups part-skim ricotta cheese (using a low-fat ricotta will reduce the fat per serving slightly)
- 6 tbs. egg substitute, divided
- 6 green onions, chopped
- 1 1/2 tsp. Italian seasoning, or add 1/2 tsp. each dried oregano, basil and parsley
- 1 10-oz. package frozen chopped spinach, thawed and excess water gently squeezed out
- 3 cloves garlic, minced or pressed
- 1/2 cup grated parmesan cheese, divided
- 2 cups grated carrots
- 1 1/2 cups (6 oz.) firmly packed grated part-skim mozzarella cheese, divided (using low-fat mozzarella will reduce the fat per serving)
- Low-Fat White Sauce (see recipe on pages 109-110)
- 1 1/2 cups bottled marinara sauce

1. Preheat oven to 350 degrees. Start boiling lasagna noodles in large saucepan until tender, then drain well. Meanwhile, spray a 9 by 13-inch baking pan with nonstick cooking spray.
2. In a medium sized bowl, blend ricotta cheese with 1/4 cup of the egg substitute, green onions, and Italian seasoning; set aside.

3. In another medium sized bowl, mix spinach with garlic, 1/4 cup of the parmesan cheese, carrots, remaining 2 tbs. of egg substitute, and half of mozzarella; set aside.
4. Make white sauce using recipe below.
5. To assemble lasagna, spread 3/4 cup of the marinara sauce over bottom of prepared pan. Lay three lasagna noodles in pan. Spread ricotta cheese mixture evenly over noodles. Spread remaining marinara sauce over the top of ricotta cheese layer. Top with three lasagna noodles. Spread spinach mixture evenly over noodles. Top with half of the white sauce. Lay remaining three noodles over the top. Spread remaining white sauce over the top and sprinkle remaining mozzarella and parmesan over the white sauce.
6. Bake uncovered in oven for 35 minutes. Let stand 10 minutes before serving.

Per serving: 375 calories, 22.5 g protein, 39.5 g carbohydrate, 14.5 g fat, 7.5 g saturated fat, 40 mg cholesterol, 4 g fiber, 705 mg sodium. Calories from fat: 35 percent.

1,252 RE Vitamin A (157 percent RDA).
16.5 mg Vitamin C (27 percent RDA).
1.8 mg Vitamin E (23 percent RDA).

Low-Fat Microwave White Sauce

Makes about 1 1/2 cups of sauce.

- 1 1/2 cups low-fat milk
- 1 1/2 tbs. butter or margarine
- 3 tbs. Gold Medal Wondra flour (quick mixing flour)
- 1/4 tsp. salt
- 1/8 to 1/4 tsp. black pepper

Mix all ingredients in a 4-cup glass measure or small glass bowl. Microwave on high for 6 to 8 minutes (or until thickened) stopping to stir every 2 minutes.

Awesome entrée recipes

 ## Power Scramble

Makes 2 servings.

- 2 eggs
- 1/2 cup fat-free egg substitute
- 1/4 cup low-fat milk
- Nonstick cooking spray
- 2 green onions, chopped
- 1/2 green, red or yellow bell pepper, chopped (or use 1/4 chopped pasilla chile pepper for a spicier version)
- 1 cup quartered cherry tomatoes (chopped Roma or vine ripened tomatoes can also be used)
- 1 cup sliced crisini mushrooms (button or other variety mushrooms can also be used)
- 1/4 cup low sodium chicken or beef broth
- 1 clove garlic, minced or pressed (or 1/4 tsp. garlic powder)
- 1 baked potato, cubed or coarsely chopped
- Black pepper (to taste)

1. Beat eggs, egg substitute, and milk with mixer until well mixed and smooth; set aside.
2. Heat a large nonstick frying pan or skillet over medium heat. Coat generously with nonstick cooking spray. Add green onions, bell pepper, tomatoes, and mushrooms to pan and cook, stirring frequently, for a couple of minutes. Add broth and garlic and cook, stirring frequently, until liquid is almost cooked off and mushrooms are tender (about 5 more minutes).
3. Meanwhile, scramble eggs as desired over low heat using a nonstick frying pan or large saucepan that has been coated with nonstick cooking spray. (Butter or

margarine may need to be added depending on the quality of the nonstick cookware.)

4. Once eggs are cooked as desired, stir in potato and vegetable mixture. Remove from heat, cover pan and let sit a couple of minutes to blend flavors. Add pepper to taste.

Per serving: 230 calories, 17 g protein, 26.5 g carbohydrate, 6 g fat, 2 g saturated fat, 210 mg cholesterol, 4 g fiber, 200 mg sodium. Calories from fat: 24 percent.

340 RE vitamin A (43 percent RDA).
78 mg vitamin C (130 percent RDA).
1.4 mg vitamin E (18 percent RDA).

 Power Quesadilla

Makes one serving.
- Canola cooking spray
- 2 flour tortillas
- 1/3 cup grated reduced fat Monterey jack cheese (or reduced fat cheese of choice)
- 2 fire-roasted green chiles (canned whole mild green chiles, such as Ortega)
- 2 green onions, chopped
- 1 tomato, sliced (discard ends)

1. Heat the nonstick medium-sized frying pan over medium-low heat. Coat pan with nonstick cooking spray. Add one flour tortilla.
2. Sprinkle grated cheese evenly over the top.
3. Split each chile in two and lay the four chile strips evenly on top of the cheese.
4. Sprinkle green onions over the top and lay tomato slices on top of that.
5. Place remaining flour tortilla on top and spray the top with nonstick cooking spray. When bottom

tortilla is lightly brown, carefully flip quesadilla over.

6. When bottom tortilla is lightly brown, remove the quesadilla to a cutting board. Cut into wedges.

Per serving: 505 calories, 23 g protein, 71 g carbohydrate, 13.5 g fat, 5 g saturated fat, 20 mg cholesterol, 4-7 g (depending on the brand of tortilla) fiber, 930 mg sodium. Calories from fat: 24 percent.

158 RE Vitamin A (20 percent RDA).
109 mg Vitamin C (182 percent RDA).
2.4 mg Vitamin E (30 percent RDA).

 Roasted Garlic and Chicken

Makes 2 servings.
- Canola or olive oil nonstick cooking spray
- 2 chicken breasts, boneless, skinless
- Black pepper to taste
- Seasoning salt to taste (optional)
- 2 tsp. olive oil
- 6 garlic cloves, peeled
- 1/2 onion, sliced thin
- 1 1/2 medium sized carrots (or 1 large), sliced thin
- 1 medium sweet potato, peeled and sliced thin
- 1 tomato, sliced
- 1 tsp. dried chervil or any other herb of choice)
- 2 tbs. dry white wine, champagne, apple juice or chicken broth

1. Preheat oven to 350 degrees. Place a 2 1/2-foot-long piece of foil in a 9" x 13" baking pan. Coat top of foil with nonstick cooking spray.
2. Lay chicken breasts in middle of foil. Sprinkle tops with pepper and seasoning salt to taste.

3. Add olive oil to small cup. Peel garlic cloves and dip in oil. Drop 3 garlic cloves evenly over each chicken breast. Lay onion slices over the chicken. Then spread carrots over the onion and potato slices over the carrots. Top with tomato slices. Sprinkle top with chervil.

4. Drizzle remaining olive oil over the top then drizzle with wine.

5. Fold foil over to wrap chicken and vegetable mixture up well. Bake for 1 hour. Cut into center of chicken to make sure chicken is cooked throughout.

   Note: To double this recipe, make two foil-wrapped chicken and vegetable packages. They will both fit in the 9" x 13" baking pan. Still bake everything for 1 hour. To serve, make sure every portion has a chicken breast, and a sampling of the various vegetables. Drizzle some of the juices over the top.

Per serving: 321 calories, 31 g protein, 33 g carbohydrate, 6.5 g fat, 1 g saturated fat, 68 mg cholesterol, 4 g fiber, 110 mg sodium (not including seasoning salt). Calories from fat: 18 percent.

1564 RE Vitamin A (196 percent RDA).
35 mg Vitamin C (57 percent RDA).
1.8 mg Vitamin E (23 percent RDA).

 # Chili Popper Casserole

Makes 4 large servings.

- 1 cup uncooked rice
- 2 cups water
- 2 tsp. canola or olive oil (optional)
- 1 15-oz. can S&W pinquitos (seasoned small brown beans), lightly drained, or use fat-free refried beans or canned pinto beans
- 1 onion, finely chopped
- 1 egg

- 2 tbsp. low-fat milk
- 2/3 cup finely ground plain bread crumbs
- 8 Ortega canned whole green chiles, mild (about 1 to 2, 7-oz. cans)
- 6 oz. reduced-fat Monterey jack or reduced-fat sharp cheddar cheese (4 oz. cut into thick slices and 2 oz. grated)
- Nonstick canola cooking spray
- 2/3 cup salsa (mild or hot depending on preference)

1. In a medium covered saucepan, start bringing rice, water and oil to a boil. Reduce heat to a low simmer, cover and cook for 15 minutes or until rice is cooked; set aside.

2. While rice is cooking, spread beans in bottom of 9" x 9" square baking pan. Top with chopped onion. Beat egg with low-fat milk in small-to medium-sized shallow bowl and set aside. Place bread crumbs in small-medium sized shallow bowl and set aside. Drain whole chiles and stuff each with cheese slices (reserve the grated cheese for garnish).

3. Start heating the nonstick frying pan over medium-low heat. Coat well with nonstick cooking spray. Using a fork or your fingers, carefully dip each stuffed chili pepper first in the bread crumbs to coat well, then in egg mixture, then in bread crumbs again.

4. Place the peppers in a frying pan. Once all of the peppers are in the frying pan, spray tops of chili peppers with nonstick cooking spray. Once the bottoms are lightly browned, flip over and cook until other side is lightly brown. Remove from pan and set aside.

5. Top beans and onion in pan with cooked rice. Spread salsa over the rice. Lay the chili peppers evenly over the salsa and top with grated cheese. Cover with foil. Bake in a preheated 375-degree oven for 25 minutes.

Per serving: 589 calories, 31.5 g protein, 92 g carbohydrate, 10.5 g fat, 5.5 g saturated fat, 76 mg cholesterol, 8 g fiber, 613 mg sodium. Calories from fat: 16 percent.

169 RE vitamin A (21 percent RDA).
73 mg vitamin C (122 percent RDA).
0.7 mg vitamin E (9 percent RDA).

 # Southwestern Chicken Casserole

Makes 6 servings.
- 4 boneless, skinless chicken breasts
- 3 cups low-sodium chicken broth
- 1 1/2 tsp. olive oil
- Nonstick canola or olive oil cooking spray
- 1 large onion, chopped (about 1 cup)
- 4 cloves garlic, minced or pressed
- 1 4-oz. can diced mild green chiles (choose medium or hot if desired)
- 1 14-oz. can ready-cut tomatoes (or chopped stewed tomatoes)
- 1 tbs. red wine vinegar
- 1 tsp. dried oregano leaves
- 1/4 tsp. pepper
- Salt to taste (optional)
- 1 15-oz. can black beans, drained and rinsed (50 percent less salt available)
- 3 cups cooked brown or white rice
- 3 cups raw finely chopped broccoli
- 4 oz. reduced fat Monterey Jack cheese, shredded (1 cup)
- 4 oz. reduced fat sharp cheddar cheese, shredded (1 cup)

1. Preheat oven to 350 degrees. Cut each breast at a diagonal into strips. Add chicken strips to medium-sized saucepan along with chicken broth. Over medium-low heat bring the broth to a gentle boil. Cover pan and reduce heat to simmer. Simmer until chicken is tender and cooked throughout (about 20 minutes). Remove chicken from broth with a slotted spoon and let cool. Once cool, cut into smaller, bite-sized pieces.

2. Heat olive oil in a large nonstick frying pan, skillet, or saucepan over medium-low heat (or spray generously with nonstick cooking spray). Add in onion, garlic, and green chiles. Cook, stirring occasionally until tender, about 4 minutes. Stir in tomatoes (including juice) red wine vinegar, oregano, pepper, and salt (if desired). Cover, reduce heat to simmer, and cook about 4 minutes. Stir in black beans and simmer 4 minutes more.

3. Coat an oblong baking dish with nonstick cooking spray. Layer rice then broccoli over the bottom of pan. Spread chicken pieces over the rice and broccoli. Top with black bean mixture. Sprinkle cheeses evenly over the top. Cover with foil and bake 30 minutes.

Per serving: 422 calories, 39 g protein, 44 g carbohydrate, 11 g fat, 5 g saturated fat, 68 mg cholestorol, 9 g fiber, 712 mg sodium. Calories from fat: 23 percent.

102 RE vitamin A (23 percent RDA).
68 mg vitamin C (113 percent RDA).
1.3 mg vitamin E (16 percent RDA).

 ## Three-Bean Power Chili

Makes 6 large servings.

- 1 tsp. ground cumin
- 1 tbs. chili powder
- 1/2 tbs. paprika
- 2 tsp. dried oregano
- 1/2 tsp. cayenne red pepper
- 1 lb. super-lean ground beef (or ground sirloin)
- 3 onions, chopped
- 2 green bell peppers, seeded and chopped
- 6 garlic cloves, minced or pressed

- 1/2 cup rehydrated sun-dried tomatoes cut into small pieces (not in oil) (Rehydrate by adding tomato pieces to small cup, cover with water, and microwave on high for about 1 minute.)
- 12 oz. dark beer or nonalcoholic beer
- 1/8 cup tomato paste
- 1 28-oz. can plum tomatoes
- 2 tbs. semi-sweet chocolate chips (optional)
- 1 19-oz. can kidney beans, drained and rinsed (1/3 less salt if available)
- 1 19-oz. can great northern beans or other white beans, drained and rinsed
- 1 19-oz. can black beans, drained and rinsed

1. Blend the spices in a small cup; set aside. In a large nonstick saucepan, over medium heat, cook and crumble ground sirloin until browned. Spoon cooked ground beef to plate and set aside.
2. Spray pan generously with nonstick cooking spray. Add onions and green pepper and cook, stirring frequently, until onions are golden brown (about 5 minutes). Stir in garlic, sun-dried tomatoes, and the spice mixture made earlier. After cooking and stirring about a minute, pour in the beer and tomato paste. Continue to cook and stir for about 6 to 8 minutes, scraping up any brown bits on the bottom of pan.
3. Stir in tomatoes and their juice, chocolate chips, ground beef, and beans and cook until chili is thick (about 45 minutes).

Per serving: 460 calories, 31.5 g protein, 67 g carbohydrate, 8.3 g fat, 2.9 g saturated fat, 20 mg cholestorol, 19 g fiber, 890 mg sodium. Calories from fat: 16 percent.

173 RE vitamin A (22 percent RDA).
69 mg vitamin C (115 percent RDA).
2.4 mg vitamin E (30 percent RDA).

Pork Tenderloins with Apples and Yams in Cream Sauce

Makes 4 servings.

- 1 pound pork tenderloin (about 2 tenderloins)
- 4 cups of sweet potatoes that have been cut into large chunks (drained canned yams can also be used)
- 1 tbs. butter
- 4 medium apples (or 3 large apples), cored and cut into 1/3-inch thick slices
- 1 tbs. sugar
- 1/3 cup apple cider
- 1/2 tbs. canola oil
- Pepper (to taste)
- 2 large shallots, chopped
- 1 tsp. dried thyme (or 1 tbs. fresh thyme)
- 1/3 cup apple or apricot brandy
- 1 cup whole milk
- 1/4 cup apple cider
- 1 tbs. Wondra (quick-mixing flour)

1. Cut each tenderloin (if small to medium sized) in half in the middle. Place one pork piece in a plastic bag and pound pork to 1/4-inch thickness using a meat mallet. Repeat with remaining pork pieces; set aside.

2. Microwave yam chunks in a microwave-safe dish with 1/4 cup of water until tender (about 10 minutes on high). Drain and set aside. Melt 1 tbs. of butter in a large nonstick skillet over medium heat. Add apple slices and let sauté for a few minutes, stirring occasionally. Pour in sugar and 1/3 cup of apple cider and continue to cook until lightly brown and slightly tender (about 5 more minutes); set aside.

3. Heat oil over medium heat in a large nonstick skillet or frying pan, spreading to coat bottom of pan. Add pork pieces and sauté until cooked through and browned (about

4 minutes per side). Season pork with some freshly ground pepper as it's cooking. Remove pork to plate and set aside. Add shallots, thyme, and apple brandy to the pan. Boil gently and briefly, scraping up browned bits from bottom of pan. Stir in milk and 1/4 cup apple cider and stir. Sprinkle 1 tbs. of Wondra over the top and stir to blend well. Boil gently until mixture thickens to a sauce consistency (just a minute or so).

4. Add yams to apples. Serve each piece of pork with a large helping of the apples and yam mixture. Spoon a generous helping of the sauce over the pork.

Per serving: 473 calories, 28 g protein, 55 g carbohydrate, 11.5 g fat, 4.5 g saturated fat, 83 mg cholestorol, 5.5 g fiber, 118 mg sodium. Calories from fat: 22 percent.

1,920 RE vitamin A (240 percent RDA).
31 mg vitamin C (52 percent RDA).
1.8 mg vitamin E (23 percent RDA).

Lemon Broccoli Chicken

Makes 4 servings.

- 1/3 cup fresh lemon juice (juice from about 3 lemons)
- 2 tbs. tequila or gin
- 3 green onions, chopped
- 2 tsp. parsley flakes (or 2 tbs. chopped fresh parsley)
- 1 tsp. dried tarragon (or 1 tbs. chopped fresh tarragon)
- 1 tsp. dried thyme (or 1 tbs. chopped fresh thyme)
- 2 shallots, chopped
- Pepper (to taste)
- 4 chicken breasts, skinless and boneless
- All-purpose flour (about 1/2 cup)
- 1 tbs. butter

- 2 cups sliced mushrooms (about 6 oz.)
- 1/2 cup + 1/8 cup whole milk (low-fat can be used but it doesn't come out quite as creamy)
- 4 cups fresh broccoli florets (about 2 broccoli crowns)
- 4 cups cooked rice

1. Add lemon juice, tequila, onions, parsley, tarragon, thyme, shallots, and pepper to a medium sized bowl. Stir to mix. Add in chicken breasts and press down on the chicken to cover tops with marinade. Refrigerate at least 4 hours (up to overnight) turning chicken once if possible. Remove chicken from marinade; reserving the marinade. Pat chicken dry with paper towels. Place some flour in pie plate. Coat chicken with flour, shaking off excess.

2. Melt butter in large high quality nonstick skillet or saucepan over medium-low heat. Add chicken and cook until brown on both sides (about 4 minutes per side. Add marinade including herbs and shallots, mushrooms and milk and bring to boil. Reduce heat to low, cover and cook until chicken is cooked throughout (about 20 minutes).

3. While chicken is cooking, microwave broccoli florets with 1/4 cup water in microwave-safe covered dish on high for about 7-8 minutes or until just tender.

4. Serve each chicken breast over a bed of broccoli and rice and drizzle a generous amount of the sauce mixture over the top.

Per serving: 510 calories, 39 g protein, 69 g carbohydrate, 7 g fat, 3.3 g saturated fat, 82 mg cholesterol, 5 g fiber, 160 mg sodium. Calories from fat: 13 percent.

186 RE vitamin A (23 percent RDA).
98 mg vitamin C (163 percent RDA).
1.1 mg vitamin E (14 percent RDA).

Sausage and Spinach Bake

Makes 6 large servings.

- 1 package (10 oz.) turkey breakfast sausage, or Louis Rich or Jimmy Dean light sausage
- 2 cups thinly sliced mushrooms
- 5 green onions, chopped
- 3 cups chopped Roma or plum tomatoes (or any vine-ripened tomato)
- 1 10-oz. package frozen chopped spinach, thawed and squeezed of excess water
- 1 tsp. dried basil
- 1/2 tsp. ground sage
- 2 cloves garlic, minced or 1/2 tsp. garlic powder
- 1/4 tsp. salt
- 1/4 tsp. pepper
- 4 oz. reduced fat Monterey jack cheese, grated (about 1 cup)
- 4 large flour tortillas (low fat brands are available in most supermarkets)
- 1 1/2 cups fat-free egg substitute

1. Preheat oven to 350 degrees. Cook and crumble sausage in a large nonstick saucepan over medium heat until nicely brown. Turn off heat and stir in mushrooms, onions, tomatoes, spinach, basil, sage, garlic, salt, pepper, and cheese.
2. Spray a 9" x 13" baking pan with no-stick cooking spray. Microwave flour tortillas on high for about 1 minute to soften (or soften by heating briefly in a nonstick frying pan.) Arrange flour tortillas to line the bottom of pan and partially up the sides of pan.
3. Spread sausage mixture evenly in pan. Top with egg substitute. Bake in oven for about 30 minutes.

Per serving: 284 calories, 24.5 g protein, 24 g carbohydrate, 10.5 g fat, 4 g saturated fat, 50 mg cholesterol, 3.2 g fiber, 740 mg sodium. Calories from fat: 34 percent.

463 RE vitamin A (34 percent RDA).
26 mg vitamin C (43 percent RDA).
1.8 mg vitamin E (23 percent RDA).

 ## Spanakopita (Greek Spinach Pie)

Makes 6 servings.

- 2 8-oz. packages frozen spinach, chopped
- 1 medium-sized onion
- 1/2 bunch fresh green onions
- 1/4 cup beer, wine, or broth
- 6 oz. reduced-fat or regular feta cheese
- 8 oz. low-fat or part-skim ricotta cheese
- 3 egg whites or 6 tbs. egg substitute
- 1/4 cup corn flake crumbs
- 1 tsp. fresh or dry dill weed
- 1 1/2 tsp. chopped garlic (or 1/2 tsp. garlic powder)
- 1 1/2 tbs. butter
- 12 sheets phyllo dough

1. Defrost spinach and squeeze out as much water as possible. In a nonstick frying pan coated with canola cooking spray, brown chopped onions and scallions in beer, wine, or both. In a medium-sized bowl, mix ricotta, feta, egg substitute, corn flake crumbs, spinach, onion mixture, dill and garlic.
2. Melt butter and get 12 sheets of defrosted phyllo dough unwrapped from box.
3. Lay 3 sheets of phyllo in a 9-inch pie plate, brushing top of each sheet lightly with melted butter. Spread

1/3 spinach mixture evenly in pie plate. Top with 3 sheets of phyllo, lightly brushing top of each sheet with melted butter. Spread another 1/3 of spinach mixture evenly in pan. Top with 3 sheets of phyllo, lightly brushing top of each sheet with melted butter. Spread remaining spinach filling in pie plate and lay the last 3 sheets of phyllo over the top, lightly brushing top side with butter. Fold all sheets of phyllo hanging out of pan back over the spinach filling and brush top with remaining butter (or spray with canola or olive oil nonstick cooking spray.

4. Bake in an oven preheated to 400 degrees for about 20 minutes (or until golden brown).

Per serving: 302 calories, 14.5 g protein, 34 g carbohydrate, 12.5 g fat, 7 g saturated fat, 37 mg cholesterol, 3.5 g fiber, 655 mg sodium. Calories from fat: 37 percent.

680 RE vitamin A (85 percent).
15 mg vitamin C (25 percent).
1.2 mg vitamin E (15 percent).

 # Tuna Cruciferous Casserole

Makes 6 servings.

- 4 cups cooked noodles of your choice
- 9 1/4 oz. can solid white tuna canned in water, drained
- 10 3/4 oz. can Reduced Fat Cream of Broccoli Soup
- 2/3 cup nonfat, light or regular sour cream
- 2 cups frozen peas with baby carrots (or similar), lightly cooked
- 4 green onions, chopped
- 4 to 6 oz. reduced-fat sharp cheddar cheese, grated
- 6 spears (uncooked) of broccoli

1. Boil noodles until tender if you haven't already done so. Drain noodles well and add to large mixing bowl. Preheat oven to 375 degrees. Coat a 2-quart casserole dish with canola cooking spray.
2. Add remaining ingredients to mixing bowl with noodles and toss to mix well. Spread into prepared pan. Top each serving with a spear of broccoli.
3. Bake for about 25 minutes (or until heated through and bubbly).

Per serving: 383 calories, 31.5 g protein, 49 g carbohydrate, 7.5 g fat, 3 g saturated fat, 61 mg cholesterol, 4 g fiber, 465 mg sodium. Calories from fat: 18 percent.

385 RE vitamin A (48 percent RDA).
156 mg vitamin C (261 percent RDA).
1.7 mg vitamin E (21 percent RDA).

 ## Carotene Chicago-Style Pizza

Makes 6 large servings.

- 2 cups canned crushed tomatoes in puree (or Italian-style stewed tomatoes, drained)
- 4 garlic cloves, minced
- 2 tbs. minced fresh basil or oregano or 2 tsp. dried
- Basic Pizza Dough (recipe follows)
- Olive or canola oil cooking spray
- 3 cups grated part-skim or low-fat mozzarella (about 12 oz.)
- 1/2 cup grated Parmesan cheese
- 2 cups assorted carotene-rich vegetables, chopped (broccoli, carrots, chile peppers, bell peppers, or spinach)

1. Preheat oven to 475 degrees. Combine the tomatoes, garlic, and herbs. Cover and set aside.
2. Press the dough over the bottom and partway up the sides of a 15-inch deep-dish pizza pan (or divide in half and press into two 9-inch cake pans). Cover with plastic wrap and let rise in a warm place for about 20 minutes.
3. Prick the bottom of the dough all over with a fork and bake for about 4 minutes. Spray the crust generously with olive oil or canola oil cooking spray. Spread the mozzarella cheese over the crust, then spoon the tomatoes on top. Sprinkle with the Parmesan cheese and then with the vegetables.
4. Bake on the bottom oven rack for 5 minutes, then move to a rack in the upper third of the oven and bake until the crust is lightly browned and the cheese is bubbly (about 30 minutes longer).

Per serving: 760 calories, 34.5 g protein, 109 g carbohydrate, 20 g fat, 8.5 g saturated fat, 37 mg cholesterol, 7 g fiber, 1,200 mg sodium. Calories from fat: 24 percent.

575 RE vitamin A (72 percent RDA).
29 mg vitamin C (48 percent RDA).
2.3 mg vitmain E (29 percent RDA).

 Basic Pizza Dough

- 1 3/4 cups warm water
- 1 tbs. sugar
- 1 package active dry yeast (1 tbs.)
- 6 cups unbleached all-purpose flour
- 3 tbs. olive oil
- 1 1/2 tsp. salt

1. Pour the water into a large bowl. Add the sugar and yeast, stir until dissolved, and let sit until foamy, about 5 minutes. When the yeast is active, stir in 1 cup of the flour.
2. Stir in the olive oil and salt. Add another 4 1/2 cups flour and mix until the dough forms a ball. Sprinkle about 1/2 cup flour onto a work surface and knead the dough until smooth and elastic, adding more flour only to keep it from being too sticky.

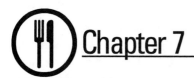 Chapter 7

Navigating the Supermarket

You may have heard the old saying that in order to eat healthy you should shop the perimeter of the supermarket. This really isn't true—there are many helpful and healthful foods you buy in the center aisles of a supermarket (and some not-so-fabulous foods around the perimeter). However, it is true that one of the most important categories of healthful food for this book (Food Steps 1-3) is usually found in that infamous perimeter—produce.

I have broken this chapter into two parts: supermarket tips for food products (which will help you follow many of the other Food Steps to Freedom) and tips for produce.

Part I: products

Don't be fooled by all the advertising slogans—not everything that says it's "healthy" or "good for you" really is. Before you purchase *anything* under the assumption of health, *read the nutrition label*. For example, you'll notice that some breads boast their "multigrain" or "seven-grain" lables...only to glance at the nutrition label to see one piddly gram of fiber per serving. Or you might see some "wheat" or "multigrain" crackers that don't even have one gram of fiber per serving.

Generally, the more you know about a food product, the better off you'll be. To begin your education, start by examining many different food labels. Start with the portion size. (What *they* think a portion is and what *you* think a portion is could be very different.) For example, some products within the same category may even have different serving sizes. Some bread labels give the nutrition information for one slice, others for two slices. Some canned baked beans and chiles give the nutrition information for a half cup, others for one cup. Then it's a good idea to just get a quick feel for the calories, fat grams, saturated fat grams, and fiber grams that product offers.

Fat-free but full of calories

Here's a newsflash: Just because a product is fat-free doesn't mean it is calorie-free or that you can eat the whole box in one sitting. In fact, many of these fat-free products have just as many calories as the full-fat versions. How can that be? In a word—sugar.

Sugar, whether it comes from honey, corn syrup, brown sugar, or high-fructose corn syrup, can add moisture and help tenderize bakery products. When added to foods such as ice cream it adds flavor and structure. I'm not surprised that manufacturers have turned to sugar for assistance while developing reduced-fat and fat-free products. Keep in mind that while a majority of the fat-free and lower-fat products on the supermarket shelves have skimmed off the fat, the calories are mostly the same as the full-fat versions (saving only 10 or 20 calories per serving).

"Fat-free" sometimes means "satisfaction-free"

Some of us may be using fat-free products as an excuse to overeat. Now, I don't think we are entirely to blame here. If these products aren't as satisfying, it's more likely that we'll eat more to become satisfied. Also, much of the advertising has *encouraged* us to eat as much as we want—after all, it's fat-free!

So what's a fat gram and calorie-watching girl to do? *Only select light and fat-free products that you truly like*—that taste satisfying to you—that you can eat in modest serving sizes. Otherwise, don't bother. For example, I really love Cracker Barrel Light Sharp Cheddar—it is real cheese to me. My family has Louis Rich turkey bacon and we don't miss the real thing. Reduced-fat Bisquick is a staple in my house. We all think Louis Rich turkey franks and Ball Park Lite franks taste terrific. These are the types of products you want to keep buying—the ones that you truly enjoy.

Some companies have gone too far

In my opinion, certain foods simply aren't meant to be fat-free. If you take all the fat out of a food that was mostly fat to begin with—such as mayonnaise, ice cream, or butter—then what have you really got? Something other than mayonnaise, ice cream, or butter—that's for sure.

More than half of the new fat-free, sugar-free, or "light" products I try end up in the garbage can. But about 20 percent (or one in five) of the products I try are keepers. A number of products have successfully found this optimal "reduced" level of fat. These are the foods that withstood a modest reduction in fat without a huge loss in taste satisfaction. You'll find them listed in this chapter.

Fiber first thing in the morning

If you eat a breakfast cereal a few times a week, you sit down to about 156 bowls of cereal a year. Whether or not you choose a whole grain cereal can make a *big* difference in the amount of fiber.

I'll tell you a secret—when you are looking down that cereal aisle in the supermarket, what really distinguishes one cereal from

Fiber in cold cerials

Cerial	Fiber(g)	Calories
All-bran Extra Fiber, 1/2 cup	13	50
Fiber One, 1/2 cup	13	60
All-Bran original, 1/2 cup	10	80
Frosted Shredded Wheat, 1 cup	10	190
100 percent Bran, 1/3 cup	8	80
Kellogg's Raisin Bran, 1 cup	8	200
Post Raisin Bran, 1 cup	8	190
Shredded Wheat 'n Bran, 1 1/4 cup	8	200
Bite Size Frosted Mini-Wheats, 1 cup	6	200
Cracklin Oat Bran, 3/4 cup	6	190
Raisin Bran Crunch, 1 1/4 cup	5	210
Total Raisin Bran, 1 cup	5	180
Bran Flakes, 3/4 cup	5	100
Complete Wheat Bran Flakes, 3/4 cup	5	90
Crunchy Corn Bran, 3/4 cup	5	90
Spoon Size Shredded Wheat, 1 cup	5	170
Mini-Wheats (Raisin), 3/4 cup	5	180
100 percent Whole Grain Wheat Chex, 1 cup	5	180
Fruit & Fibre (Dates, Raisins, Walnuts), 1 cup	5	210
Grape Nuts, 1/2 cup	5	210
Raisin Nut Bran, 3/4 cup	5	200

another is not its fat and sodium content, but sugar and fiber content. Some have a lot more sugar and these are usually the cereals that have a lot less fiber too. In the table on page 130, you will find most of the cereals available with five grams of fiber or more per serving. If you are wondering where the Cheerios and whole grain Wheaties are, they only contain three grams of fiber per serving—they didn't make the cut.

Fiber where you least expect it: supermarket surprises

	Fiber (g)	Calories	Fat (g)	Sodium (mg)
Breads* (# slices)				
Oroweat Light 100-Percent Whole Wheat (2)	7	80	0.5	N/A
Oroweat 100 Percent Whole Wheat (2)	4	180	2	N/A
Oroweat Bran'nola (2)	4	180	2	N/A
Oroweat Best Three Seed (2)	4	200	7	N/A
Oroweat Best Winter Wheat (2)	4	240	6	N/A
Oroweat Bagels, 100 percent Whole Wheat (1 bagel)	9	240	1.5	N/A
Oroweat Bagels, Health Nut (1 bagel)	5	270	4.5	N/A
Oroweat Bagels, Oat Nut (1 bagel)	4	270	4	N/A
Iron Kids, Fiber-Fortified White (2)	4	160	2	N/A
School Bus, Fortified White Bread (2)	3	170	1	N/A
Crackers & other bread products				
Triscuit Reduced-Fat (8 crackers)	4	130	3	170
La Tortilla Factory 100 percent Whole Wheat Tortilla (1 tortilla)	9	60	0	180
Canned Bean Products (1/2 cup)				
Taco Bell Vegetarian Refried Beans	8	140	2.5	500
Ortega Refried Beans	9	130	2.5	570
Ortega Fat-Free Refried Beans	9	120	0	570
Rosarita Low-Fat Black Refried Beans	5	90	0.5	460
Rosarita Vegetarian Refried Beans	6	100	2	500
B&M Original Baked Beans	6	170	2	380
S&W Chili Beans Zesty Sauce	6	110	1	580
S&W Santa Fe Beans	6	90	0.5	680
Hormel Vegetarian Chili With Beans	3.5	100	0.5	390
Dennison's Turkey Chili With Beans	3.5	105	1.5	535
Frozen Foods				
Gardenburger, Veggie Burger (Patty Only), 2.5 oz.	4	130	3	290
Eggo Nutri-Grain Multigrain Waffles, 2	5	160	5	360

*These above bread products usually contain around 400 milligrams sodium per 2 slice serving.

Sweet tooth selections

Choose...	Instead of...
• Starbucks Frappuccino (Mocha) Frozen coffee bar (1 bar = 120 calories, 2 g fat)	• 1/2 cup Starbucks Coffee Almond Fudge Ice Cream (250 calories, 13 g fat)
• Ben & Jerry's Chocolate Fudge Brownie Low-fat Frozen Yogurt (1/2 cup = 190 calories, 2.5 g fat)	• Fudge Brownie a la mode (350 calories, 20 g fat)
• Reduced-Fat Chips Ahoy (3 cookies = 140 calories, 5 g fat)	• Chunky Chips Ahoy (3 cookies = 240 calories, 12 g fat)
• Snackwells Mint Crème cookies (2 cookies = 110 calories, 3.5 g fat)	• Mystic Mint cookie or mint ice cream (2 cookies = 180 calories, 9 g fat)
• 3 Reduced Fat Oreo cookies with a glass of 1 percent low-fat milk (230 calories, 6 g fat)	• Cookies & Creme ice cream (1 cup) or a cookies & creme candy bar (ice cream = 350 calories, 24 g fat)
• Jell-O Instant Chocolate Pudding (Made with 2 percent milk) (1 serving = 160 calories, 2.7 g fat)	• Chocolate cream pie (1 small slice = 305 calories, 16 g fat)
• Betty Crocker Low-Fat Fudge Brownie Mix (1/18 pan = 130 calories, 2.5 g fat)	• Regular Fudge Brownie (1/18 pan = 175 calories, 9 g fat)
• Strawberries or other berries with 1/2 cup light vanilla ice cream (145 calories, 3.3 g fat, plus 1.3 g fiber)	• 1/2 cup ice cream (about 250 calories, 13 g fat)
• Lemon or coconut meringue pie (1/8 pie = 240 calories, 8 g fat)	• Lemon or coconut cream pie (1/8 pie = 415 calories, 22 g fat)
• Mrs. Smith's Blackberry Cobbler (1/8 cobbler = 250 calories, 9 g fat)	• Mrs. Smith's Berry Pie (1/12 pie = 330 calories, 15 g fat)
• 1 piece angel food cake with 1/2 cup berries or other fruit (175 calories, <1 g fat, plus 4 g fiber)	• 1 thin piece frosted cake (275 calories, 12 g fat)

Sweet tooth selections, continued

Choose...	Instead of...
• Weight Watchers Smart Ones New York Style Cheesecake with Black Cherry Swirl (150 calories, 5 g fat)	• Frozen Mixed Berry Swirl New York Style cheesecake (1/8 pie = 340 calories, 19 g fat)
• One-crust pies (pumpkin, fruit tarts) (1/12 of Sara Lee Pumpkin pie = 173 calories, 7 g fat)	• Two-crust fruit pies (1/12 pie = 330 calories, 15 g fat)
• Mini scoop of key lime pie sherbet (1/4 cup = 60 calories, 1 g fat)	• A slice of key lime pie (400 calories, 26 g fat)
• Mini scoop of raspberry sorbet (Haagen Daaz brand) (1/4 cup = 55 calories, 0 g fat)	• 1/2 cup of gourmet raspberry truffle ice cream (or similar) (290 calories, 20 g fat)
• 1/2 cup flavored strawberry or lemon yogurt blended with 1/2 cup and 1/4 cup light Cool Whip (180 calories, 4 g fat, plus 1.5 g fiber)	• 1 thin slice of lemon or strawberry mousse cake fruit (260 calories, 14 g fat)

Shopping with a sweet tooth

If there is a dessert you really want, please enjoy it. People can refrain from overeating favorite foods if they give themselves the special foods they want from time to time. For all the days in between, here are some simple ways to cut some extra calories in the dessert department. (See the table on pages 132-133 for more information).

Dessert can also be a great way to enjoy fruits. You'll notice many of the suggestions above give you ideas on how to include fruits.

Frozen entrées

I have found there are two types of people—people who seek out frozen entrées, and people who avoid them like the plague. However, frozen entrées can come in handy in many

Frozen entrées

	Calories	Fat(%*) (g)	Fiber (g)	Sat. Fat(g)	Sodium (mg)
Frozen Pizza					
DiGiorno Four Cheese Pizza (1/3 of a 12 ounce pizza)	280	9(29%)	2	5	700
Wolfgang Puck's Mushroom & Spinach Pizza (1/2 of a 10.5 oz. pizza)	270	8(27%)	5**	3	380
Wolfgang Puck's Four Cheese Pizza, 1/2 of a 9.25 ounce pizza	360	15(37%)	5	6	530
Three-Cheese Oreida Bagel Bites (4 pieces)	190	6(28%)	1	3.5	530
Healthy Choice					
Chicken Enchiladas Suiza	280	6(19%)	5	3	440
Shrimp & Vegetables	270	6(20%)	6	3	580
Herb Baked Fish	340	7(19%)	5	1.5	480
Traditional Breast of Turkey	290	4.5(14%)	5	2	460
Chicken Enchilada Suprema	300	7(21%)	4	3	560
Lean Cuisine					
Chicken w/ Basil Cream Sauce	270	7(23%)	3	2	580
Chicken in Peanut Sauce	290	6(19%)	4	1.5	590
Baked Fish w/ Cheddar Shells	270	6(20%)	4	2	540
Fiesta Chicken (with black beans, rice, and vegetables)	270	5(17%)	4.5	5	90
Cheese Lasagna w/ Lightly Breaded Chicken Breast Scaloppini	290	8(25%)	3	2	590
Shrimp & Angel Hair Pasta	290	6(19%)	1	1	590
3-Bean Chili	250	6(22%)	9	2	590
The Budget Gourmet					
Three Cheese Lasagna	310	12(35%)	2	6	700
Fettucini and Meatballs in Wine Sauce w/ Green Beans	270	7(23%)	3	3	560
Marie Calender's					
Chili & Cornbread	540	21(35%)	7	9	2,110
Sweet & Sour Chicken	570	15(24%)	7	2.5	700

Frozen entrées, continued

	Calories	Fat(%*) (g)	Fiber (g)	Sat. Fat(g)	Sodium (mg)
Marie Calender's, continued					
Beef Tips in Mushroom Sauce	430	17(36%)	**6**	7	1,620
Turkey w/ Gravy and Dressing	500	19(34%)	4	9	2,040
Spaghetti and Meat Sauce	670	25(34%)	**9**	11	1,160
Stuffed Pasta Trio	640	18(25%)	**5**	9	950
Swanson					
Mexican Style Combination	470	18(34%)	**5**	6	1,610
Chicken Parmigiana	370	17(41%)	4	5	1,010
Herb Roasted Chicken Breast Tenders w/ Rice & Vegetables	310	7(20%)	3	2.5	780
Turkey Dinner	310	8.5(25%)	**5**	2	890

*Percent of calories from fat
**Bold and underlined type denotes that fiber content equals five grams or higher

situations—as a quick lunch during the workweek and as an easy dinner if you live alone or with one other person. I usually have a frozen pizza on hand in case of a meal emergency. (I've included frozen pizza information too.)

The problem with frozen entrées is this: The ones that are lower in fat are almost always too low in calories and carbohydrates and meager in the vegetable department. Many contain around 300 calories—the amount of calories in one measly bagel. In order to make the entrées more nutritious and satisfying, you might consider adding fruits and vegetables. You might even need to add some cooked rice, noodles, or even some grated cheese.

Some frozen entrées are brimming with sodium and others aren't that bad (check the table above) and you'll see what I mean. If you need to watch your sodium intake, keep an eye on this portion of the nutrition label.

The case for canola oil

Over the past few years, canola oil has been keeping olive oil company on the great oil pedestal. Olive oil has some phytochemicals that canola oil doesn't have. But there are some things that canola oil has that olive oil doesn't. Here are the four main things canola oil has going for it:

1. Canola oil (and olive oil) are high in monounsaturated fats, the preferred type of fatty acids when it comes to improving blood lipid levels and helping prevent heart disease and some cancers.
2. Canola oil is a plant source of EPA—an omega-3 fatty acid. Omega-3 fatty acids have been linked to lowering both blood pressure and serum triglyceride levels, preventing blood clots, and possibly increasing HDL(good cholesterol-levels). The two cancers that omega-3s may help prevent are colon and breast cancer. Some plant foods contain alpha-linolenic acid, which the body can partially convert to the omega-3 fatty acid, EPA.
3. Canola oil is generally higher in vitamin E than some other common vegetable oils. Canola oil contains about nine IU (or less) per tablespoon.
4. Canola oil works out well in cooking and baking because it has a neutral taste and is stable at high temperatures.

Convenient high monounsaturated fat sauces

I have listed some store-bought sauces below. In order to qualify they *had* to contain canola or olive oil (our high monounsaturated fat oils). The marinara/spaghetti sauces listed below are the only ones that sit on the shelf at room temperature—and they are pretty good. You can always add in your own super lean ground beef, mushrooms, garlic, onion, and other spices if you want to dress them up a little. The rest of the sauces can be found either in the frozen food section (next to the frozen raviolis) or in the refrigerated fresh pasta section.

However, what they all have in common is that they are a godsend to the busy weekday cook. Just open a tub or a bottle

Healthful red sauces (1/2 cup sauce)

	Calories	Fat(sat.)	Fiber	Sodium
Five Brothers				
Grilled Eggplant & Parmesan	100	3(.5)	3	540
Grilled Summer Vegetable	80	3(0)	3	550
Mushroom & Garlic Grill	90	3(0)	3	550
Marinara w/ Burgundy Wine	90	3(0)	3	480
Classico				
Tomato & Basil	50	1(0)	2	390
Fire-Roasted Tomato & Garlic	60	1(0)	2	390
Sutter Home				
Italian Style w/ fresh onions and herbs	80	2(0)	4	520
Barilla				
Green and Black Olive	80	2.5(.5)	3	1,010
Roasted Garlic & Onion	80	3.5(0)	<1	460
Mushroom & Garlic	70	2(.5)	3	610
Tomato & Basil	70	1.5(.5)	3	640
Marinara	70	2(.5)	2	430

Healthful pesto sauces (1/4 cup sauce)

	Calories	Fat(sat. fat)	Sodium
Contadino Reduced-Fat Pesto with Basil	230	18(4)	560
Armanino˙ Roasted Bell Pepper Pesto	140	14(2)	350
Armanino˙ Pesto	190	18(3)	370
Armanino˙ Dried Tomato & Garlic Pesto	210	17(1.5)	210

˙Armanino Foods Of Distinction, Inc. Hayward, CA 94544

and pour it in. How easy it that? The tomato-based sauces will also contribute those helpful phytochemicals found in cooked tomato products.

Healthful Salad Dressings and Spreads

	Calories	Fat	Sat. Fat	Sodium
Mayonnaise (1 tablespoon)				
Safeway Select Real Mayonnaise w/ canola	100	11	1	80
Spectrum Canola Mayo	100	12	1	80
Spectrum Lite Canola Eggless Mayonnaise	35	3	0	60
Salad dressing (2 tablespoons)				
Kraft "Special Collection"				
Sun Dried Tomato	60	4.5	0	330
Italian Pesto	70	5.5	2	60
Balsamic Vinaigrette	110	12	1	290
Kraft "Light Done Right"				
Red Wine Vinaigrette	50	4.5	0	330
Italian	50	4.5	0	230
Raspberry Vinaigrette	60	4	0	270
Cucumber Ranch	60	5.5	4	80
Catalina	80	5	0	400
Kraft				
Roasted Garlic Vinaigrette	50	4.5	0	270
Caesar Parmesan	60	5	1	450
Newman's Own				
Dynamite Lite Italian	45	4	0	370
Balsamic Vinaigrette	90	9	1	350
Bernstein's				
Italian Cheese & Garlic	110	11	1	340
Red Wine & Garlic Italian	110	11	1	250
Parmesan Garlic Ranch	140	14	1	300
Balsamic Italian	110	11	0.5	270

High monounsaturated fat salad dressings and spreads

The products on page 138 exclusively contain canola oil, olive oil, or a combination of the two (mostly monounsaturated fat). Most of us use these ingredients almost on a daily basis. Switching to a different product is an easy way to increase the amount of monounsaturated fats we are taking in. Compared to saturated and polyunsaturated fat-laden products, I can vouch that most of the following products taste great. I wouldn't use them if they didn't.

Part II: The most powerful produce

When it comes to all the nutrition advantages to eating lots of fruits and vegetables, I don't know where to start. Well, I guess we could start with fiber, phytochemicals, vitamins, and minerals. We could then look at their low amounts of calories, fat, saturated fat, or cholesterol. This is all very powerful stuff. However, take a look at this: Women who never ate carrots or spinach had twice the risk of getting breast cancer compared to women who did eat them more than twice a week (*Cancer Epidemiology, Biomarkers & Prevention*, November 1997). Now this is *very* powerful stuff. Researchers are still learning about the power of produce and the way it influences our health and various diseases, but we know enough to say that fruits and vegetables in general are a big part of a healthy, well-balanced meal. And we know that certain fruits and vegetables appear to have higher levels of vitamins, minerals, phytochemicals, and other important components that make them particularly helpful. To find out more about these, keep reading.

How to increase the antioxidants in your diet

- Go for the **green**. Kale and spinach are two top antioxidant-rich veggies. Other top greens are collard

Antioxidant-rich plant foods

	beta carotene	vitamin C	vitamin E
Fruits			
Cantaloupe, 1 cup cubed	✓	✓✓	
Grapefruit, half (or 1/2-cup of sections)		✓	
Guava, half		✓✓	
Kiwi, 1		✓✓	
Mango, half or 1/2-cup slices	✓	✓	
Orange, 1 (or 1 cup of sections)		✓✓	
Papaya, half or 1 cup slices		✓✓	
Strawberries, 1 cup whole or sliced		✓✓	
Tangelo, 1		✓	
Tangerine sections, 1/2 cup		✓	
Vegetables			
Beet greens, boiled, 1 cup	✓	✓✓	
Bell pepper (red or yellow), 1/2 whole		✓✓	
Broccoflower, 1 cup cooked		✓✓	
Broccoli, 1 cup raw or cooked		✓✓	
Brussels sprouts, 1 cup cooked		✓✓	
Butternut squash, 1 cup bakedcubes	✓✓	✓	
Carrot, 1/2 cup steamed		✓✓	
Cauliflower, 1 cup raw or cooked		✓✓	
Chili peppers, 1/4 cup raw or canned	✓	✓✓	
Chinese cabbage, 1 cup steamed		✓✓	
Dandelion greens, 1 cup boiled or 2 cups raw	✓✓		
Dock/sorrel greens, 1 cup raw	✓	✓✓	
Green pea pods, 1 cup cooked		✓✓	✓
Hubbard squash, 1 cup baked	✓✓		
Kale, 1 cup boiled	✓✓	✓✓	✓
Kohlrabi, 1 cup boiled		✓✓	
Mustard greens, 1 cup boiled	✓	✓	
Peas, 1 cup raw		✓✓	
Pumpkin, 1/2 cup boiled	✓✓		
Snow peas, 1 cup steamed		✓✓	

✓ **Food servings providing at least 50 percent of the RDA.**
✓✓ **Food servings providing around 100 percent of the RDA.**

Antioxidant-rich plant foods, continued

	beta carotene	vitamin C	vitamin E
Vegetables, continued			
Spinach, 1 cup boiled	✓✓		
Spinach, 2 cups fresh chopped	✓	✓	
Sweet potato, 1 baked or 1/2-cup canned	✓✓		✓
Swiss chard, 1 cup boiled	✓	✓	
Turnip greens, 1 cup boiled	✓✓	✓	
Winter squash, 1 cup cubes or 1/2 cup mashed	✓		
Yams, orange, 1/2 cup mashed	✓✓		
Beans and bean products			
Lima beans, 1 cup cooked		✓	
Soybeans, 1 cup cooked			✓✓
Soybeans, 1/2 cup roasted		✓	
Tofu, 1/2 cup			✓
Nuts			
Almonds, 1 ounce			✓✓
Filberts/hazelnuts, 1 ounce	✓		
Sunflower seed kernels, 2 tablespoons roasted			✓✓

✓ Food servings providing at least 50 percent of the RDA.
✓✓ Food servings providing around 100 percent of the RDA.

greens, Swiss chard, or mustard greens. And one bright green fruit—kiwi—also packs an antioxidant punch.

- **Cruciferous family** vegetables are brimming with antioxidants and phytochemicals. In addition, research is going on now to test the cancer protective properties of plant compounds found in the cruciferous vegetables for their ability to lower cancer risk. Choose Brussels sprouts, broccoli, cauliflower, or cabbage.
- Find the **orange** and you'll find carotenoid-rich produce. Include sweet potatoes, cantaloupe, carrots, winter squash, pumpkins, or apricots.

Fruits and vegetables rich in carotenes

	beta carotene	lutein/ zeaxanthin	lycopene
Fruits			
Apricots	✓		✓(dried)
Cantaloupe	✓		
Guava or guava juice			✓
Mangoes	✓		
Pink grapefruit			✓
Watermelon			✓
Vegetables			
Bok choy	✓		
Broccoli	✓	✓	
Brussels sprouts		✓	
Carrots	✓		
Fennel	✓		
Green leaf lettuce		✓	
Greens: beet	✓		
Collard	✓		
Mustard	✓	✓	
Kale	✓	✓	
Leeks		✓	
Peas		✓	
Pumpkin	✓	✓	
Red pepper	✓		
Romaine lettuce	✓		
Spinach	✓	✓	
Squash, butternut/acorn	✓		
Summer squash		✓	
Sweet potatoes and yams	✓		
Swiss Chard	✓		
Tomatoes (red) tomato sauce and tomato paste			✓
Winter squash	✓		

- Are you seeing **red**? Red-colored produce, that is. They are rich in antioxidants. Try strawberries, raspberries, blueberries, blackberries, plums (and prunes), tomatoes, red grapes (and raisins), red peppers, or cherries.
- Don't forget the **citrus family** of fruits, famous for being rich in vitamin C: oranges, grapefruit, lemons, or limes.

Follow the yellow (dark green and red) brick road

Foods rich in the antioxidant-rich carotene family (which includes the well-known beta carotene) have been linked to helping protect against different types of cancer. Although there are thought to be 500 different members of the carotene family, let's look at the four that scientists suspect help prevent disease:

- **Beta carotene.** This antioxidant may reduce risk of some cancers by protecting cells from damage. (Tends to be found in orange or deep yellow and dark green vegetables.)
- **Lutein/zeaxanithin.** These compounds may help protect against macular degeneration, a leading cause of blindness in older people. (Tend to be found in dark green vegetables.)
- **Lycopene.** Lycopene has been linked with a decreased risk of prostate cancer. (Tends to be found in red or pink fruits and tomato products.)

 Chapter 8

Restaurant Rules to Live By

I'm getting the distinct impression that most people don't cook anymore. I write a national column called *The Recipe Doctor*, where I "doctor" recipes people love to make. This being said, I can't tell you how often people confess to me, "I love your column...but I don't cook." I am amazed that people can enjoy reading a column about cooking when they don't use the recipes or don't cook at all.

Often the people telling me they don't cook are people with young children. So I have to wonder. If all these people aren't cooking, what are they eating? Most of us could guess the answer to that question. For many the answer is "fix-it" foods such as frozen entrees, hot dogs, macaroni and cheese from a box, and restaurant and fast-food fare.

What's the fallout from eating out?

A large portion of Americans eat out at least one meal a day, which means restaurant and fast-food fare probably contributes to at least one-third of their daily calories. From a fiscal point of view, Americans spend about 42 percent of our food budget on eating out. Whichever way you look at it, the bottom line is that many of us eat out every single day. What effect has all this eating out had on our nutritional intake? Let's not even get into the grams of fiber or vitamins and minerals that are going unconsumed due to our eating out splurges—let's just focus on how our daily calories and fat grams are being affected.

Wouldn't you guess that our calories and fat grams tend to go up the more we eat out? According to a recent study that's exactly what happens.

Restaurants: an opportunity to eat healthy

Restaurant dining is no longer a special occasion—it's just part of our normal busy day. This means we have to rethink the way we view restaurant dining. It isn't an opportunity to splurge anymore—it needs to be an opportunity to eat healthy (at least most of the time).

The problem with healthy dining is that just about everything is working against it. Everything about eating out screams "indulge, indulge, indulge!" Many restaurants use saturated fat and lots of it, the menu choices are too tempting to pass up, and portion control is next to impossible. Besides all that, at restaurant prices you want to get your money's worth (which usually means a meal you really enjoy in impressive portions). So how do you balance all this with health? It's all in your attitude.

When eating and feeling healthy becomes your focus, you still want to get what you pay for in restaurants. It's just that what you want is a meal that will contribute to improving (not destroying) your health. Surely, fancy restaurants can prepare some dishes per your request. In fact, more and more restaurants are offering healthful options on their menu.

Of course you do have to be willing to give this healthy restaurant fare a try. Many casual dinner chain restaurants like Applebee's, Bennigan's, and Chili's do have "lite" selections on their menus, but judging the platters of burgers and ribs I saw passing by when I was there last, it isn't the healthy choices being ordered by most.

What if you have just one higher-fat menu item? Make sure the rest of your meal is healthy and light. Part of the trouble with restaurant meals is that we simply don't know how to quit while we're ahead. What do we do typically? We eat a high fat appetizer (such as buffalo wings). Then, we chase that down with a high-fat entrée (such as a burger or a creamy pasta dish). Then, we pair that with something equally as fatty (such as french fries or garlic bread)...only to top the meal off with a very rich dessert. If we just stuck to one high-fat choice and made healthier choices to go with it, we would be a lot better off.

When eating out, there are two things we need to keep in mind: how to keep from eating too much fat, saturated fat, and calories and how to eat more fruits, vegetables, and whole grains. To help you do that, take a look at some dining do's and don'ts.

Dining "do's"

- **Do order entrees or side dishes bursting with greens or other high-nutrient vegetables and whole grains when possible.**
- **Do make every bite count.** Don't hurry through your meal but rather savor each bite. Restaurant food is usually prepared with extra care, quality, and attention to detail.
- **Do focus on eating when you are hungry.** If you are hungry an hour or more before you are due to eat out, go ahead and eat something. Satisfy your hunger with a little something such as a piece of fruit or a quick grain product (such as cereal, some wheat crackers, etc.).

- **Do stop eating when you are comfortably full.** This is tough in a restaurant but try to listen to your tummy (not your eyes or your wallet). When your stomach is comfortable and you no longer feel hungry, stop eating. If you can, take your leftovers home or back to the office refrigerator so you can have the rest later when you are hungry again.
- **Do try and choose restaurants that you know make great tasting, healthy dishes.**
- **Do prepare to hear comments and questions from coworkers or family.** You might hear "Are you on a diet?" Just reply, "No, this is just the way I like to eat."
- **Do order a steak, a piece of pie, or anything else you really want...every once in a while.** If you don't have your favorite restaurant foods every now and again you'll start feeling deprived. That can lead to, among other things, a bad attitude.
- **Do ask the server how something is prepared.** You can ask:

    What cut of meat is used? The leaner choices are flank, tenderloin, sirloin, London broil, eye of round, top and bottom round and sirloin tip.

    What type of fat is used in this dish? You can ask that olive or canola oil be used instead of other oils (and in some cases, in place of butter).

    Is this dish served with sauce or added butter? Ask that the butter be left out or the sauce served on the side. This way you can decide how much you need.
- **Do ask that they take the chicken skin off before the dish is prepared.** More than half the fat in poultry is in and around the skin (most of it being saturated fat) and dark meat has about double the fat of white meat. Not that dark meat is bad—you also get more iron and other nutrients for your trouble. Just make sure and take the skin off if you can—to at least

shave off some fat grams and calories. Of course all of this skinning isn't going to do you much good if your skinless breast or thigh is then fried. Frying can increase the fat two- to five-fold (depending on whether it is battered then fried).

- **Do ask for substitutions or special preparations.** Three out of five restaurant managers surveyed by the National Restaurant Association were willing to make substitutions in ingredients when asked. Besides, the worst they can say is "no."

- **Do enjoy grilled, steamed, or broiled seafood in restaurants.** When prepared without a lot of extra fat, seafood is a wonderful restaurant choice. It is something we tend not to make for ourselves at home. Even the fattier fishes compare in total fat and calorie content to the leaner steaks. And many seafood selections are a great source of omega-3 fatty acids and other important nutrients.

- **Do choose the leanest steak available when you feel like eating steak.** Instead of a prime rib, order a leaner steak (such as a sirloin or a filet mignon). Try it with in-season vegetables and a baked potato with a tablespoon of sour cream and you're in business.

- **Do feel free to enjoy a green salad with your meal.** Go heavy on the beans, tomatoes, vegetables, and spinach leaves and light on the croutons, bacon bits, chopped egg, cheese and dressing. Choose a dressing made with olive or canola oil when possible.

- **Do order the dressing on the side when you order a Chicken Caesar or Chinese Chicken Salad.** The full-fat dressing does most of the damage with this dish. Drizzle around two tablespoons over the top of this big salad.

- **Do start your lunch or dinner with wonderful clear soup** (such as minestrone, Manhattan clam chowder, or chicken noodle). Creamy soups tend to be loaded with fat and calories. If you want creamy soup, opt for a cup instead of a bowl.

- **Do enjoy roasted vegetables with your meal.** Roasted vegetables are becoming quite the latest thing in restaurants and cooking magazines. The roasting brings out wonderful flavors. Usually if oil is used on the vegetables, restaurants opt for olive oil.
- **Do enjoy a baked potato with your meal.** Just go light on the butter and sour cream. One pat of butter or margarine and one-eighth cup of sour cream will usually do the job. Each pat (or teaspoon) of butter adds about 35 calories and four grams of fat. One-eighth cup of sour cream adds 60 calories and six grams of fat. Add the baked potato and you've got a grand total of 315 calories, 10 grams fat (28 percent calories from fat), six grams saturated fat, 23 mg cholesterol, and five grams fiber.
- **Do share a dessert you really want with friends at the table.** I know what it is like to see that dessert cart glide past with what seems like all your favorite desserts. Ordering a fancy dessert everyday isn't a good idea, but every once in a while you should enjoy sampling a dessert, especially if you are sharing it. If there is something that really appeals to you but you are comfortably full from the meal, order it to go and you can nibble on it later when you are hungry again.
- **Do seek out bean dishes.** We all need to get in the habit of eating more beans, which are bursting with nutritional attributes. Beans aren't something most families make at home. This makes them the perfect dish to order in restaurants. You'll find bean dishes at Mexican, Southern, Italian restaurants, as well as some Indian and Asian ones.
- **Do ask that your stir-fried dishes at Chinese restaurants be used with only a little oil.** Stir-fried dishes are lower in fat than deep-fried dishes (steamed dishes are lower in fat than stir-fried dishes). But many Chinese restaurants will go easier on the oil—all you have to do is ask. Even fried rice can be made with a

lot less oil. You might also want to ask that the flavor enhancer MSG be left out if it bothers you.

- **Do enjoy those fancy grilled chicken sandwiches (but watch out for the company your grilled chicken is keeping).** These sandwiches are often served with bacon, cheese, and mayonnaise—all of which bump up the fat grams and calories a lot. When you can, enjoy the grilled chicken breast with lettuce, tomato, onion, mustard, or barbecue sauce instead.

- **Do order chicken, shrimp, or vegetable fajitas instead of steak fajitas.** Not including the sour cream or guacamole, a typical steak fajita entrée adds up to 31 grams of fat (12 grams are saturated).

- **Do order the tofu or vegetarian version of some of your favorite Chinese dishes.** This is an easy way to eat more tofu and vegetables. If you like chow mein, order vegetable chow mein. If you adore curry chicken or moo shu chicken, order curry tofu or moo shu tofu.

- **Do seek out Mediterranean restaurants.** There are so many health attributes of Mediterranean cooking— the use of olive oil is well known. But perhaps even more important is their use of fish and vegetables.

- **Do enjoy French fries at home.** You can buy the lower- fat frozen seasoned variety and bake them in the oven. They taste great, without all that fat from deep frying.

- **Do enjoy higher-fat condiments in small quantities.** I know butter, margarine, salad dressings, mayonnaise, whipped cream, sour cream, or cream cheese taste great. But a little goes a long way. Keep it that way.

Dining "don'ts"

- **Don't skip meals earlier in the day as a way of "sav- ing up" calories for when you eat out.** This only makes you over-hungry (which leads to overeating) and over-ordering. It's always important to eat when you are hungry and stop when you are comfortable.

- **Don't eat a large or high-fat lunch on a workday.** It will fill your stomach and leave you feeling sluggish and sleepy for hours. Keep working lunches modest in size and fat grams. You are more likely to have the energy to go back to work and get a lot done.
- **Don't feel like you have to order something from each menu category (appetizer, entrée, salad, and dessert).** Think about what you really want to eat and how much food you are going to be comfortable eating.
- **Don't be fooled.** Sometimes dishes that sound healthy are served with sauces or added butter. This can turn a broiled chicken breast or piece of fish into the nutritional equivalent of a marbled steak.
- **Don't order those third- or half-pound burgers with all the extras.** Go for the quarter pounders and dress them with mustard, ketchup, barbecue sauce, lettuce, onion, or tomato instead of bacon, cheese, or creamy sauces.
- **Don't order deep fried foods often.** Not only are these dishes high in fat and calories, but restaurants tend to use oils other than olive and canola oil to do their frying.
- **Don't have more than one of those appetizers "you just gotta have."** In other words, if you *must* have buffalo wings, potato skins, and fried mozzarella sticks—have one (or two) wing, skin, or stick and be done with it. They are all so high in fat and calories that much more than that will add up way too quickly.
- **Don't overdo the alcohol.** Some restaurants are set up to get you to order as many drinks as possible. To keep alcohol in check, ask for water along with your drink. Order nonalcoholic beer, wine, and mixed drinks (this will cut calories by more than half.) If you are going to have an alcoholic beverage, have it with your meal. Buy wines by the glass, not the bottle.

- **Don't go heavy on the sauces...unless it is a marinara (tomato-based) sauce.** If you do end up ordering an entrée that comes with a cream sauce, try to enjoy the dish with only a few tablespoons (or one-eighth cup) of the sauce.
- *Definitely* **don't eat a big dinner.** As Americans, we tend to eat our biggest meal at the end of the day (especially if we are out at a restaurant)...but that doesn't make it right. It's a bad habit we have gotten into.

  I know this may sound ridiculous but you can use the palm of your hand to give you an idea of the serving of meat you should be eating. This is about three to four ounces (depending on the size of your palm).

Takeout taxi time

Is eating take-out from restaurants healthier than eating fast food? We better hope so—more and more people are doing it. The number of meals eaten at home but prepared elsewhere has almost doubled over the last decade. And even the "white-tablecloth" type restaurants are getting into the act, with about 75 percent of them offering food to go (about 90 percent of family restaurants do). Here are some of the top takeout options:

- **The pizzeria.** Two little slices (or one big one) of authentic Italian pizza with tomatoes, basil, garlic, and cheese. Order it topped with whatever veggies you wish. Add a big green salad made at the restaurant or at home (don't forget a scoop of kidney or garbanzo beans) and dress it in light dressing. Other possible entrees include pasta marinara, mushroom spaghetti, or tortellini with marinara sauce. Go ahead and sprinkle some freshly grated Parmesan over the top—a tablespoon only adds 28 calories and 1.9 grams fat, and five milligrams cholesterol for all that flavor.
- **Chinese take-out.** Curry chicken or tofu with vegetables or shrimp and vegetable stir-fry over steamed rice can be

a pretty good option—especially if you ask for the cook to go light on the oil. Other good options are chicken, tofu, or vegetable chow mein (light on the oil) and vegetable lo mein (with soft noodles). The vegetables you often see in Chinese dishes—cabbage, bok choy, carrots, and broccoli—are high in phytochemicals and other promising anticancer compounds. Oh, and don't toss the fortune cookie. Each one adds only 30 calories.

- **Rotisserie.** Go for those moist, delicious slices of freshly carved rotisserie turkey breast. Add a side of new potatoes, in-season vegetables, and maybe a little dish of hot cinnamon apples. You can substitute roasted chicken breast for the turkey if need be (just try to take the skin off). Other good choices are a meatloaf sandwich (no cheese please), a lean ham sandwich with mustard or cranberry sauce (hold the mayo), or homestyle chicken noodle soup with a roll or a wedge of corn bread.

- **Burrito bar/fresh Mex.** Depending on how adventurous you want to be, these burrito bars offer everything from roasted tofu and vegetable burritos to veggie or bean burritos (go for the whole pintos or black beans). All can be made on your choice of a spinach, white, or wheat tortilla (the latter of which contributes about nine grams of fiber alone). Throw in your mild, hot, or smokin' salsa and call it a healthy lunch. Even if you opt for the chicken or steak burritos you can't get in too much trouble...as long as the burrito isn't deep fried or filled with lots of cheese, guacamole or sour cream. Just remember—a dollop will do ya. Other good choices are soft chicken tacos, chicken fajitas, or chicken enchiladas (going light on the cheese and sour cream).

What? No nutrition label?

Obviously, restaurant meals don't usually include nutrition labels like supermarket products. Sometimes, if there are "healthy fare" or "light menu" options, the restaurant may have the nutrition information for those items included on the menu or in a pamphlet somewhere. But mostly it is nutritional pot luck—we have no clue how many calories, grams of fat, or saturated fat we are about to partake of.

So if you want to make healthier choices we basically have to follow some general suggestions (like those in the previous "do's and don'ts" list) and then hope for the best. If you make pretty healthy choices, emphasize vegetables, and eat when you are hungry and stop when you are comfortable—the calories and fat grams will be in the dietary ballpark.

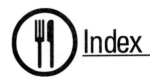 Index

abortion, induced, 15
acetaldehyde, 33
alcohol intake, 27
alcohol, 6, 13, 22, 26, 33, 46, 52, 71-72, 83, 151
alpha carotene, 27
alphalinolenic acid, 29
alpha-linolenic acid, 66
American Cancer Society, 7, 17, 19, 20
American Institute for Cancer Research, 9, 10, 19, 20
amino acids, 40, 41
antioxidants, 26, 27, 28, 47, 52, 62, 65, 85

B vitamins, 55
bacon, 39
barbecuing, 39
BCRA gene mutations, 14
beans, 28, 29
beta carotene, 27, 40, 41, 50, 52, 53, 143
body fat, 26, 81
body mass index, 27
body water, 81

bone density, 81
bones, 13, 19, 24
Brazil nuts, 24, 63
BRCA1, 13
BRCA2, 13
bread, 41
breakfast, 86
breast cancer
    and diet, 22-35, 36
    and dietary fat, 24, 29-31
    and HRT, 15-16
    death rates of, 7
    detection of, 16
    factors contributing to, 10
    family history of, 10, 13, 27
    getting, 9
    increased risk of, 10
    invasive, 11, 27
    possible warning signs of, 16
    rates and geography, 14
    recurrence of, 10, 71
    risk and age, 11
    risk, reducing, 10
    spread of, 13
    stages of, 18
    treatment of, 19

breast self-exams, 7
breast tissue, fibrocystic, 10
breastfeeding, 14

caffeine, 11, 40
calcifications, 20
calcium, 85
caloric intake, 74
calories, 128
    burning, 85
    counting, 80
cancer cells, 7
cancer development, stages of, 12
cancer,
    bladder, 33
    cervical, 51
    colon, 24, 36, 37, 53, 55, 68, 71
    digestive tract, 33
    esophagus, 33
    gastrointestinal tract, 40
    growth, 40
    larynx, 33
    liver, 32
    lung, 6, 33, 53, 68
    mouth, 33
    ovarian, 5
    pharynx, 33
    prostate, 24, 36, 37, 51, 68
    rectal, 24, 33, 36, 51, 68
    skin, 6, 53
    uterine (endometrial), 24, 25, 26, 68
carbohydrates, 26
carcinogens, 12, 34

carotenoids, 26, 27, 41, 46, 50, 53
cell division, 12
change, stages of, 88-89
chemotherapy, 19
chest wall, 19
childbearing, 14
chlorogenic acid, 39
chocolate, 11, 31
cholesterol, 62
cigarette smoke, 26
    exposure to, 15
clinical breast exam, 16, 18
constipation, 55
cooking oils, 69-70, 135-136, 147
corn oil, 25
cysts, 15

dairy, 31, 77
desserts and sweets, 130, 132-133, 149
diabetes, 80, 82
diet, 9, 10, 13
dieting, 74, 82
DNA, 12, 24
    damage to, 26
ducts, 20

eating habits, 75
eating out, 144-154
eggs, 24, 35, 63
energy level, 24
estrogen, 14, 15, 18, 20, 25, 26, 31, 32, 33, 34, 37, 54, 72

exercise, 6, 13, 46, 75, 76-78, 85, 87

fat, 23, 46, 67-69
  amount of, 30-31
  monounsaturated, 69-71
  saturated, 22, 31
  types of, 31
  unsaturated, 22
fat-free products, 128-129
fatty acids, 35
FDA, 7
fiber, 26, 32, 46, 53, 54-57, 75, 83, 85, 128-129, 131
fibroadenomas, 15
fibrocystic breast disease, 11
fish oil, 23
fish, 35, 41, 68, 71
flavonoids, 53
flaxseed, 6, 23, 29, 65, 71
folic acid, 53, 62, 72
free radicals, 26, 52
frozen entrées, 133-135
fruits and vegetables, 22, 23, 24, 26, 27, 29, 31, 32, 39, 40, 42-43, 45, 46-50, 56, 83, 85, 139-142
  number of servings of, 28, 47
  ways to eat more, 48-49
fruits, citrus, 51

garlic, 23, 29
genes, 13, 18
genetics, 6, 8, 73
  mutation, 13

testing, 14
grilling, 39, 40, 68

heart disease, 5, 6, 7, 16, 29, 68
heart, 24
heat, 26
heterocyclic amines (HCAs), 40, 68
hormone replacement therapy (HRT), 15, 19, 20
hysterectomy, 17

immune system, 33, 70
indole-3-carbinol, 51
insulin, 82
intestines, 32
isoflavones, 34, 37, 38, 64

lean meats, 24
legumes, 24, 26, 56, 63
leukotrienes, 70
lignins, 28, 29, 55, 62, 65
lipids, 26
liver, 13
lobules, 20
low-sodium diet, 11
lumpectomy, 20
lumps, 11, 13, 16
  benign, 18
  precancerous, 11, 15
lungs, 13, 19
lutein/zeaxanithin, 27, 143
lycopene, 143
lymph nodes, 7, 18, 19

mammogram, 7, 16-18, 67
  baseline, 17
  frequency of obtaining, 17
mammography, 16
mastectomy, 20
  modified radical, 5
mayonnaise, 138
meat, 31, 46, 63
  marinating, 68
menarche, 27
menopause, 6, 8, 10, 13, 14,
  16, 18, 37, 38, 73, 77, 80
menstrual cycle, 11
menstruation, 8, 10, 14, 17
metabolism, 40, 81, 86
methylselenol, 24
milk-producing glands, 18
minerals, 26, 55, 85
miso, 39
motivation, 89
muscle mass, 81
muscle strength, 81

nitrosamines, 33, 39
nutrition labels, 127-128

OB/GYN, 7
obesity, 7, 14, 34, 46, 74
occupation, 10
oil seeds, 29
omega-3 fatty acid, 29, 31, 35,
  66, 68, 70, 71, 76, 85
omega-6 fatty acids, 25, 31,
  70, 71
omega-9 fatty acids, 85

oncogenes, 20
oral contraceptives, 15
osteoporosis, 7, 16, 81
overweight, 6, 13
oxidation, 51-52

palpate, 20
P-coumaric acid, 39
pectin, 53
perimenopause, 15
pesticides, 42-43
pesticides, exposure to, 15
phenolics, 55
phenotic acids, 37
phytate, 55
phytic acid, 37, 55
phytochemicals, 25, 26, 51, 85
phytoestrogens, 34, 37, 53, 55
phytosterols, 62
plant sterols, 55
pollutants, 10, 26
Polycyclic Aromatic
  Hydrocarbons (PAHs), 40
portion sizes, 86, 87
poultry, 35, 41, 68
pregnancy, 25
  intake of fats during, 15
premenopause, 27-28, 64
produce, 26, 42, 139-143
  organic, 43
prostaglandins, 70
protease inhibitors, 36, 55, 62
proteins, 26, 44
psychological assistance, 14

radiation, 19
radon, 10
recipes, 91-126
    entrée, 110-126
    pasta, 106-109
    salad, 91-98
    soup, 98-106
red meat, 68, 147
renal disease, 80
risk factors, 8, 14, 15
    known, 6, 13
    suspected, 6, 13

salad dressings, 138
saponins, 55, 62
saporins, 36
sauces, 136-137
seafood, 24, 63, 148
secondhand smoke, 52
seeds, 28
selenium, 24, 26, 41, 52,
    62-63
self-exam, 11, 16, 18
    when to perform, 17
sentinel node biopsy, 7
smoking, 9, 52
snacking, 83
soluble fiber, 29
soy, 23, 34, 36-37, 38, 64
soy milk, 38
soybeans, 26, 29, 36, 38, 71,
    85
stem cells, 20
strength training, 81-82
sugar, 128
sun, exposure to, 9, 52

supplements, vitamin and
    mineral, 41-42, 47

takeout, 152-153
Tamoxifen, 20
tea polyphenol, 25
tea, 25
tempeh, 38
tobacco, 7, 10, 33
tofu, 38, 64, 150, 152
trans fatty acids, 31
tumors, 7, 16, 30, 32, 34, 40,
    67, 70, 71, 72
    speed of growth, 18
Type II diabetes, 7

ultraviolet light, 26

vegetables, cruciferous, 51
vitamins, 26, 85
    vitamin A, 26, 27, 33, 52
    vitamin B-12, 85
    vitamin B-6, 62
    vitamin C, 26, 27, 31, 39,
        40, 41, 51, 52, 53
    vitamin D, 77, 85
    vitamin E, 26, 27, 33, 35,
        39, 41, 42, 52, 53, 55, 76

weight gain, 34
wheat fiber, 32
whole grains, 22, 24, 26, 28,
    29, 32, 56, 63, 85
whole wheat, 55

X-rays, 10, 13, 26

zinc, 85